'In this short compendium, Liz Rot
In account after account, the m
and lessons learned rise from the
the faces, feel the pain, the pride,
have spent the better part of the l
of pandemic anxiety and grief an _ ...o.... cuents suffering
unspeakably complicated bereavement. Remarkable in its plainspoken
eloquence and critical commentary, this book captures the panoramic
impact of the global crisis as revealed in the lives of the healthcare workers,
teachers, immigrants, youth and families who have "weathered the storm".
I recommend it to anyone compassionate, curious or concerned enough to
dive deeply into the experience of trauma and resilience, tissues in hand,
and open to cultivating a fuller humanity.'
Robert A. Neimeyer, editor of *The Handbook of Grief Therapies* **and
Director, Portland Institute for Loss and Transition, US**

'The Covid pandemic is already becoming the subject of much
reinterpretation over time. Covid is now the stuff of myths and legends
for politicians and scientists in their autobiographies and books, and
there is a lot of revisionism too. This is why the accounts in this book of
'ordinary people' whose voices have gone largely unheard are invaluable.
Looking forward, the real challenge is to ensure our parliament commits
to new legislation that will rebuild and reinstate services to safeguard the
public health against future pandemics.'
**Allyson Pollock, clinical professor of public health, Newcastle University,
and former member of Independent SAGE**

'This important book reminds us that the deaths caused by Covid
pandemic were not simply a national tragedy and a scandalising testimony
to incompetent and corrupt government; most of all, they were deeply
personal instances of love and loss. We need texts like this to tell the truth
about the pandemic. Health and social care workers and the other essential
workforces held up their side of a public service obligation to put people
first, while politicians shamefully served their own interests, with fatal and
long-term debilitating consequences. These workers are the true heroes of
our times, and for far too many this recognition has to be posthumous.
When we fail to learn the lessons of history, we are undoubtedly condemned
to repeat egregious mistakes. We must do so much more than merely clap
for carers. If we are to weather future storms, we must assertively defend
and bolster the NHS and wider welfare systems.'
**Mick McKeown, professor of democratic mental health and member
of Unison's National Nursing and Midwifery Sector Committee**

'As we who have survived emerge from our places of shelter and safety in the aftermath of the Covid-19 pandemic, we must confront our losses and reflect on life itself and reasons to go on. Liz Rothschild's book provides us with the reality of others' experiences, the sharing of which allows us the opportunity to further reflect on how devastating a time we have all endured. Above all, these powerful accounts provide us with a sense of self, of how precious life is, and how we must continue to survive for those whom we've lost. This is an immensely emotional and extremely important book.'

Sonia Winifred, psychodynamic psychotherapist and supervisor, CBT practitioner and local councillor, London Borough of Lambeth

'These stories take us to the epicentre of UK citizens' experiences of Covid. Liz Rothschild has simply asked people what happened to them, and here are the truths. I am impressed by her torch shining into dark corners to seek out those not expecting to be asked. It is a harrowing, compelling and uplifting read, reflecting the Covid years in a carefully crafted and digestible way. Professionally or anecdotally, this book is a must-read. Long Covid is put out on the table as a main course, not as an unpleasant left-over. The prevailing attitude to education, public health and the way our young people have been affected is clearly and strongly described; the commentaries are intelligent and helpful. The inclusion of individual artwork and poetry lifts us into that healing sphere of imagery and imagination, while the personal reflections are inciteful and heart-felt. This is a very important book in the context of the re-evaluation of the pandemic.'

Jo Bousfield, community theatre director, writer, and part of the Good Grief Project – www.thegoodgriefproject.co.uk

'At a time when the truth about the pandemic is so contested, it's a relief to find here a multiplicity of different personal stories, all speaking their truths, even as they sometimes contradict each other. How refreshing to hear from the bus cleaner as well as the doctor; from the child suffering with long Covid as well as the teacher. As any storyteller knows, a story can only unfurl itself fully when the listener is attentive. Liz Rothschild has clearly listened well, and the result is a satisfying collage – each voice and each chapter offering colour and contrast in relation to the others. As we begin to look back on the pandemic and look forward to what comes next, this compassionate collection of stories will help us to hold more of the diversity and complexity of what we collectively experienced.'

Jackie Singer, storyteller, musician and author of *Birthrites: Rituals and celebrations for the child-bearing years*

WEATHERING THE STORM

STORIES OF LOVE, LIFE, LOSS AND DISCOVERY IN THE TIME OF COVID

EDITED BY LIZ ROTHSCHILD

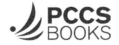

First published 2023

PCCS Books Ltd
Wyastone Business Park
Wyastone Leys
Monmouth
NP25 3SR
UK

Tel +44 (0)1600 891509
contact@pccs-books.co.uk
www.pccs-books.co.uk

This collection © Liz Rothschild
Illustrations © the artists

All rights reserved.

No part of this publication may be reproduced, stored in a retrieval system, transmitted or utilised in any form by any means, electronic, mechanical, photocopying or recording or otherwise, without permission in writing from the publishers.

The authors have asserted their right to be identified as the authors of this work in accordance with the Copyright, Designs and Patents Act 1988.

Weathering the Storm: Stories of love, life, loss and discovery in the time of Covid

British Library Cataloguing in Publication Data.
A catalogue record for this book is available from the British Library

ISBNs   paperback 978 1 915220 25 7
          epub 978 1 915220 26 4

Cover design by Jason Anscomb
Printed in the UK by Severn, Gloucester

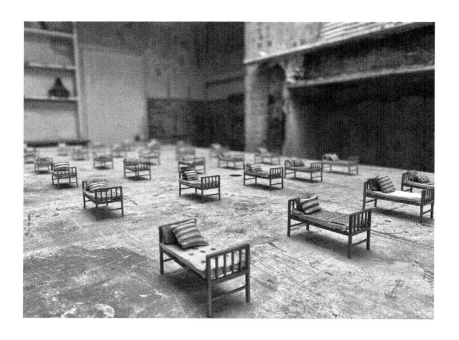

Weathering the Storm:
Stories of love, life, loss and discovery in the time of Covid

Contents

List of illustrations

Acknowledgements

I am so grateful to my keen-eyed editor, Catherine Jackson, at PCCS Books for her skill at editing and her understanding support throughout. It has been a pleasure working with her again. She directed me towards Dr Lynne Gabriel and Dr John Wilson at York St John University. Their blend of academic research with running a regular therapeutic group for people bereaved by Covid-19 meant they were able to get permission for a number of the stories in the 'Torn Apart' chapter. In approaching the 'On the Frontline' chapter, I knew I wanted to broaden out the understanding of where that frontline was and who were the key workers, but clearly the medical profession was central to those stories, and I am indebted to Dr Jo Withers, who put me in touch with a significant number of people working in many different medical fields. I am grateful to Patrick Vernon, Razia Aziz from Waytu and Anita Luby from the Death Positive Library network, among others, for using their networks to spread the word about my need for stories from the global majority. The chapter 'Our Future' contained a narrow range of experience until expert commentator Jo Holmes put me in touch with Gordon Knott at Croydon Drop-in Centre, and he was key to providing some of these narratives with promptness and sensitivity. Rose-Anne O'Hare sought out stories from those she has worked with over the years as a bereavement counsellor. Clare Davis, whose artwork is also featured in this book, was generous with her contacts with people living with disabilities and, with Alison Giraud-Saunders (who led me to Sam Clarke at Disability UK), ensured there was better representation from those communities. I was also very well supported by Kodama Allende, who as well as sharing her own story tracked down other contacts and information for me for the chapter on 'Long Covid', as well as contributing her own commentary. Judith Emmanuel was generous with her contacts in Manchester, widening the age range and background of participants included.

And, as always, thanks to my family and friends for bearing with my preoccupation with 'the book', and my daughter, son and partner for offering cogent and loving advice about its shortcomings while there was still time to remedy them.

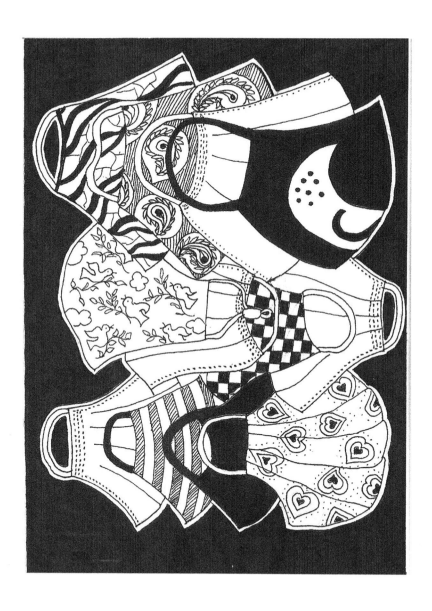

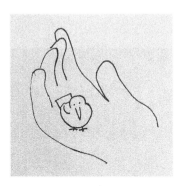

Dedication

'Those who tell stories survive'
From *Burntcoat* by Sarah Hall (Faber & Faber, 2021)

Every single person in the world has their own story about the pandemic. This book captures a few of them. It is an act of remembering, of honouring, of discovery and of survival. In deep gratitude to all those who entrusted me with their stories.

The royalties from the sales of this book will be shared with Southall Black Sisters and Long Covid Support.

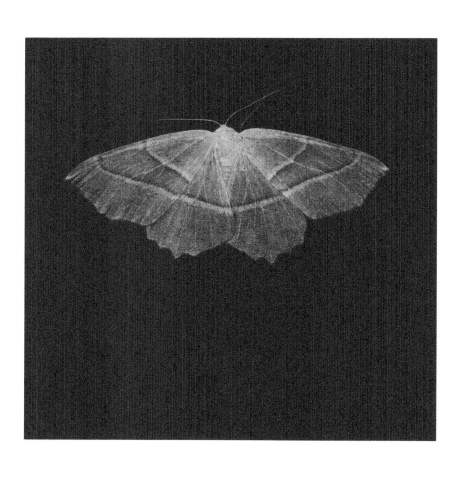

Introduction

Liz Rothschild

Do you remember when you first began to grasp how serious this all seemed to be? Already the beginnings of it begin to fade and blur. For me, it was when I went to shop at my local supermarket and, for the first time, saw those circles on the ground outside and everyone standing apart from one another. We were all wearing a variety of different masks; one looked very sinister indeed, with two filters on either side, rather like a World War II gas mask. Everyone was silent. We stood there, anxiously wondering what to do with the shopping when we got it home and whether we would find what we needed in the supermarket – hovering in that freshly discovered liminal place between trust and risk.

Finally, after we had stood for some time like this, I turned to the person behind me and said, 'It looks like we are going to be here for some time. We might as well talk to each other.' We started to share our concerns, what we had heard on the news and by hearsay, and then the person in front of me joined in too. Other conversations began further down the queue. It felt as if we had broken a spell that had been keeping us apart.

'Fear' and 'frightened' were probably the words I heard most often from people when gathering the stories in this book. Laura Dodsworth has written extensively about how fear was promoted as a means of controlling us in the UK, in her book, *A State of Fear* (2021). When fear is rife and we are told to isolate, we become removed from the comfort of our shared humanity. I hope these stories will remind us just how essential to our wellbeing that connection with each other is. The stories in the media of people stockpiling loo rolls are far outweighed by those that reveal the prevailing decency and bravery of human beings.

Quite a few people have been saying to me recently, 'Your work has got really relevant now, hasn't it?' I am a performer, a celebrant, and I run a green burial ground. I am also passionate about death education. They mean this very sincerely – as if death goes in and out of fashion and I am suddenly right on trend. I know what they are referring to, of course: a lot of the time we can push our mortality to the edges of our vision, until sudden death or illness forces it centre-field. The pandemic has made our vulnerable mortality all too plain and in a uniquely isolating way. With that has come much pain and suffering, but also other revelations. My fervent hope is that we will take note of what the pandemic exposed about the inequalities in our society *and* what makes life worth living.

This book emerged out of my previous collection, *Outside the Box: Everyday stories of death, bereavement and* life, which PCCS Books published in 2020. The book went to print too soon for me to be able to include anything of substance about the effects of the Covid-19 pandemic, and I simply added a postscript noting some of the key impacts we were becoming aware of at the time, such as the enforced separation and the use of technology to try to bridge the gap. The plan was to add another chapter at the reprint stage. That expanded into this book, which is similarly grounded in my belief that, when we share our stories, we become less isolated and gain a wider perspective.

The process of gathering the stories has been different this time. In the earlier book, most of the stories came to me as a result of my work and through touring my show, *Outside the Box – A Live Show about Death*. I gathered well above 400 stories from my audiences – touching, funny, angry and informative. The stories reflected those audiences – predominantly female, white, middle class and middle-aged or older – perfectly mirroring me. This time I began with a blank sheet of paper – no live performances and just an idea for themes, which changed somewhat as I went deeper into the territory. I knew I had to find networkers who would help me extend the range of people I could reach, and I am indebted to many people who trusted this project and helped it become richer and more challenging and reflective of our society. I list and thank them fully in my acknowledgements. All the stories, with a couple of exceptions, are drawn from the United Kingdom, and 98% of the storytellers were directly in touch with me.

When we tell and listen to each other's stories, our worldview broadens and we remember how interconnected we are. Stories are my bread and butter – simple, comforting and nourishing.

Weathering the Storm is divided into six chapters, each ending with an expert commentary giving a broader context to the topic, drawing out themes and offering deeper insight into what is being described. Each chapter is also rounded off with a resource list offering the reader further information, resources and sources of support. Inevitably, because humanity is anything but tidily compartmentalised, a number of stories could have been located in several of the chapters, and the choice of which came down to a fairly arbitrary decision. It is a book that can be read consecutively or dipped into. It's up to you.

Chapter 1, 'On the Frontline', features stories from the many people who continued to work in frontline positions, some acknowledged, like doctors, nurses and emergency services, and others who were largely ignored and invisible – cleaners, bus drivers, shopworkers, delivery drivers, teachers and social workers, to name a few.

The second chapter, 'We Are Not All in the Same Boat', contains stories from many different communities who were disproportionately impacted by the pandemic. It was notable that some people living in more socially deprived circumstances chose not to emphasise this aspect of their experience in what they wrote. There is still shame in speaking publicly about this kind of deprivation. So, you will see that this aspect is often made more explicit in the accounts of those whose jobs involve working with them. Richard Wilkinson and Kate Pickett's seminal book *The Spirit Level: Why greater equality makes societies stronger* (2009) documents and evidences the corrosive impacts of inequality on people's lives, education, opportunities and mental and physical health. The impact of the pandemic underlined their findings with stark brutality.

Chapter 3, 'Torn Apart', documents the impact of Covid on how people died, funeral procedures and the acute isolation of the grieving processes that followed. In Chapter 4, 'Our Future', children and young people, crucially, speak for themselves and bring their own insights and considerable wisdom. This chapter also includes the voices of adults who worked with them, bringing their professional perspective. The experiences of the pandemic were very different for the different generations and that needs to be recognised. Chapter 5, 'Long Covid', gives voice to adults and children struggling with the continuing effects of the virus, finding themselves having to fight to get their condition acknowledged and understood, and learning how to help each other.

The final chapter felt very important to include and is called 'Emerging'. It is about the positive discoveries people made during the pandemic. It is subdivided into 'Community stories' and 'Personal change stories', as a lot happened in both these categories. It is not an easy chapter to read, perhaps, if you feel your life was destroyed by what happened to you during the pandemic, but to me it says so much about human beings and how we build, or rebuild, resilience.

Two stories about vaccination appear in two different chapters. I have chosen not to give particular weight to the highly contentious debates about vaccination – they are not relevant to the book's themes and aims. Nor have I included any narratives from those who believe Covid-19 was some kind of government (or other) conspiracy, because I cannot see any evidence to support this.

Some excellent books have already emerged on Covid-19 and its impact, but they mainly cover the experience from a medical perspective (see the resources for 'On the Frontline'). However, there are now a number of fictional accounts, such as *Summer,* by Ali Smith (2020). This book differs from them all in that it presents a multi-faceted and, therefore, at times contradictory picture of this period, from many different perspectives.

Numerous longitudinal studies will be carried out, reports will be written and, as I complete this book, the government enquiry has finally opened. In-depth comparisons with other countries will also be valuable in helping us learn from the experience. Over time, we may be able to draw clearer conclusions about how the pandemic was handled. This book does not attempt this kind of analysis. It presents the lived experience. What is unavoidable is the conclusion that the experiences we went through were often at odds with the public messaging coming from government, as chillingly revealed in several of the stories in 'On the Frontline' and 'Torn Apart'. We do not have to wait for the outcome of all the reports and enquiries to know where some of our attention at least needs to be focused.

I hope you feel inspired by the stories you read here, and that some, at least, touch on your own experiences. I would love to hear from you if you want to share a story about an important theme you feel has not been told here, or to offer any other feedback. You can contact me at the email address below.

Liz Rothschild
Westmill Woodland Burial Ground
tour@fullcircleproductions.org.uk

August, 2022

References

Dodsworth, L. (2021). *A state of fear: How the UK government weaponised fear during the Covid-19 pandemic.* Pinter & Martin.

Rothschild, L. (Ed.). (2020). *Outside the box: Everyday stories of death, bereavement and life.* PCCS Books.

Smith, A. (2020). *Summer.* Penguin.

Wilkinson, R. & Pickett, K. (2009). *The spirit level: Why greater equality makes societies stronger.* Bloomsbury.

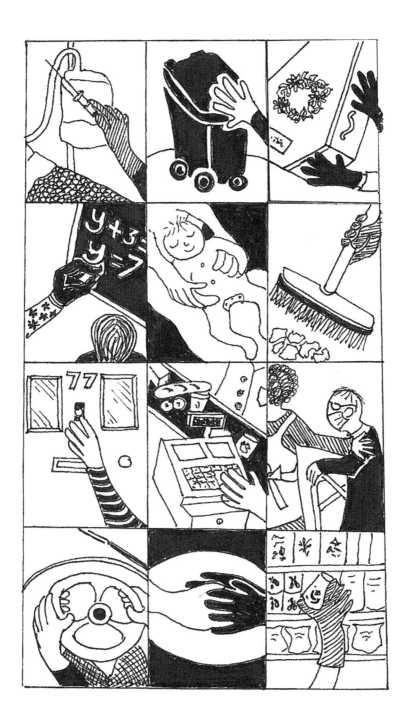

1.

On the frontline

She wanted to come home

Julie Kay, Wirral Older People's Parliament

My neighbour, I'll call her Cindy, went into hospital for gastric investigations, and was diagnosed with cancer. She caught Covid in hospital and her cancer prognosis was not good, and she wanted to come home. Home was unfortunately not fit. Her daughter had to clean and clear the ground floor before Cindy could be discharged. Her daughter doesn't drive, and they could not afford night-time care. I offered to do this, as emergency back-up, and to go in during the day with PPE on. As a nurse, I realised Cindy didn't have long left, and one early morning the carer found her peacefully passed away. Had she not come home, this would have been a very different experience for her and her daughter because of the extremely damaging hospital restrictions that were in place, which in my view were unnecessary during palliative care.

https://wirralopp.co.uk

It shouldn't have been like that

GP trainee

I am a currently a GP trainee. I originally intended to be a surgeon but the surgical recruitment I applied for was cancelled because of Covid and I couldn't keep waiting for jobs to become available. So my life has had to totally change direction. And I feel lucky to still have work. To have a routine. To feel I can be useful.

During the first lockdown, I was doing locum work in a sarcoma unit. It was very sad to see patients coming in with very advanced symptoms. Due to Covid, they had not come forward for investigation or their appointments had been cancelled, so by the time they presented to us it was quite late. Patients who could potentially have had treatment were too advanced. We could only give them a diagnosis, knowing they had very little time to adjust to what was happening to them. I remember particularly one young man in his early 20s. It shouldn't have been like that.

And then there were the mothers. During the second lockdown, as I'd started my GP training, I was attached to a paediatrics unit. I was quite excited. I thought, okay it's not surgery but I will get to be with all these new mums and their babies. It wasn't like that. We couldn't spend too much time with the babies to limit the risk of infection. Do what you have to do and go. No chatting, no admiring the baby. It was so hard for the parents. The dads at first could only be there for the birth, then they had to go. Later they could come in for one hour a day. One hour is not enough when you are coping with a new baby. The mums were in their bays or rooms. They could not help each other or even talk much. Everyone was scared. New mums, mums who'd had Caesareans, mums with twins. Each of them facing everything alone. I remember crying mum after crying mum. The wards awash with emotion. It was so hard for the midwives and all the staff. There was this feeling of helplessness. Nothing more you could do to help them. It took its toll.

Did I do enough?
Junior doctor

I am one of the cohort of students that was rushed into hospitals before we had completed our training. This is the story I have chosen to tell. It was the end of the longest run of night shifts I hope ever to have to endure. Despite my best efforts, three of the four patients I'd spent the most time with had died: a young man with Down's syndrome, a father in his 50s and a frail grandmother. The fourth, a lady in her 50s, was hanging on following a catastrophic haemorrhage. It had been a totally surreal nightmare. The floor of the whole corridor near the patient's side-room was covered in blood. I resembled an axe murderer but was still trying to encourage the (now barely conscious) patient.

The registrar poked her head around the door and said, 'You've done enough, let's get croissants.' I still don't know if that lady survived, I was too exhausted and scared to find out. My almond croissant was like ash in my mouth. The most devastating part of trying to care for sick patients through the pandemic wasn't actually the reduced support available with so many staff sick, or the fact that everyone was burning out. It was the fact that patients were suffering, fearing for their lives, and sometimes dying so very alone in the hospital. As a doctor, I was often the only human contact they had in the face of death. Keeping professional boundaries in your head, in that situation, was hard. I often got home feeling like a complete failure.

They were not alone
Julia Parker, Shout volunteer

I am trained to listen, understand and support anyone in their darkest moments. We are a texting service, and the majority of those who contact us are young people, but as the waves of Covid-19 hit, I could see I was having a deluge of conversations with frontline workers of all ages. Desperate doctors and nurses unable to see a way to cope with the inhuman demands on their energy and time and their apparent inability to prevent seriously sick people from dying. Overwhelmed, shattered healthcare workers shared words to the effect of: 'I'm meant to save people, but I don't know how to save myself.' Pre-pandemic, I would wait five or 10 minutes for a conversation to come in. By December 2021, there was always a queue of 50, 100, 200 people waiting for us to offer the support they so desperately needed and deserved. It was challenging. It was draining. It was relentless. But simultaneously it wasn't actually about the numbers; it was about being there, in the moment, for each individual person. They were not alone in facing desperate situations and I felt humbled to be able to help them work towards a calmer place.
https://giveusashout.org

At arm's length
GP to a care home

At the start of the pandemic, I was personally looking after a large care home whose patients mostly had dementia, as well as assisting in the care of patients in other nursing homes in the practice area. The initial move of patients untested for Covid out into vacant nursing home beds produced a problem that many nursing homes were not prepared for. It was frustrating being the visiting GP yet having no control over the actions of an independently run and staffed nursing home as the decisions regarding how to isolate possible cases of Covid, avoiding the mixing of patients (especially those with mental health difficulties) and use of PPE had to reside with the management of the home. Despite the best of intentions and efforts by stressed care home staff, many of whom rapidly suffered Covid themselves at an early stage, there was an inevitable loss of life among the residents. Along with this, a distance suddenly appeared between the care home and the surgery, with fewer, shorter visits and much more remote working. Conversations with relatives were suddenly more at arm's length and the work felt much less personal and satisfying. My personal opinion is that, post-lockdown, the return to the more traditional and supportive role of primary care will be slower as we first struggle to re-balance our day-to-day relationships with patients in the surgery.

He didn't sign up to be in danger

Leshie Chandrapala

My dad always wanted to be a bus driver. He was very committed to his job, very professional. He always arrived on time. He never took a day off sick. He was the guy you could always rely on. Always there for everyone. He was 64. He had no underlying health conditions, he ate very healthily, and he died of Covid. We thought if he got Covid he would recover. I was asking him all the time, 'How are you at the garage? Are you protected? Are they limiting the numbers on the buses?' He said, 'Don't worry, I'm fine.' He thought it was very important he kept driving his 92 bus as it took people to Ealing Hospital. That was where he died in the end.

When he finally got to hospital, they said he was very sick and put him on a CPAP machine on a Covid ward, but he wasn't getting enough oxygen. So then they took him to the ICU, and he ended up on a ventilator. A chasm opened up in my heart. I thought, 'This is really bad', and that was the start of a really lonely journey. Then they took him off the ventilator and we had to say goodbye via Facetime. I don't know if he heard us. I hope so. I was calling on the universe to give me strength.

I am so angry he was not protected. I have heard from his colleagues that they were not being properly looked after. They asked us to bring his hearse past the bus garage. He was a very charismatic man. Hundreds of them lined the streets. Grown men and women weeping openly. I will never forget it. Dad was a key worker. He was told his job was vital. His death was a workplace death. When he signed up to be a bus driver, he did not sign up to be in danger. It is not like joining the army. And he did not shy away from the danger when it came. I want answers from Transport for London and the Ministry of Transport. I want accountability. I want to know why the recommended measures were not put in place by the garage. I am so glad I have joined others in Covid-19 Bereaved Families for Justice. Each of us have different fights and we support one another. It is hard work grieving and even harder to grieve and campaign at the same time.

I clean the hospital like I clean my home
Hospital cleaner

I am from Goa and live in Swindon with my husband and three children. I enjoy working at the hospital. I like working as a cleaner, meeting many patients, and I enjoy sharing their stories and mine with them. I was worried about catching Covid but got used to it and was happy to continue working. I have not had Covid. I have been vaccinated. We had enough supplies of the right sort of PPE and were taught how to 'don' and 'doff' the PPE properly. I felt supported by my managers.

It was frightening to see how many people there were in hospital with Covid, especially during the first wave. I felt as though my work made a difference and patients and relatives spoke their appreciation and said I was doing a good job. The patients felt reassured with the cleaning happening. I felt safe at work during Covid. I had no experiences of fear or anxiety among the staff. I felt guilty when I was cleaning a patient's room wearing PPE and sorry for them as they had to see me dressed up like that because they were ill. I also didn't feel good in front of the patients as they might think I was covering up because they were 'sick'. I felt sorry for them because they had Covid and I thought it must be scary for them. I used to ask the patients how they were feeling.

I used to worry about going home from work and changed my clothes before I left the hospital. Straight away when I got home, I would go in the shower. My family were worried about me going to work during the first lockdown but didn't try to stop me. My husband used to just say, 'Take care'.

The hospital is my second family, so I am not afraid. I clean the hospital like I clean my house and take pride in my work. Thank you for giving me the opportunity to speak about this.

Moral injury
Paramedic

I am a part-time paramedic with the London Ambulance Service. My abiding memory of 2020 is of fear. Our fear and the fear of the people we were attending to. There was no vaccine and we were going into houses without adequate PPE. Each shift, we would have to borrow from the hospital or return to base when we had run out and hope the team leaders had managed to find some stock for us. We are used to handling death and cardiac arrest and horrible accidents, but they do not endanger us. I rarely go home from a shift without having had some kind of abuse, but I can press the panic button and help arrives pretty quickly. There is no panic button you can press to remove the threat of Covid.

I did not have to work but I felt I owed it to my colleagues and the country to do what I could. We handled it with our usual black humour. But some things get to you. Normally, we assess a patient and give them a national early warning score based on their life signs. If it is five or above, we blue light them into the hospital resus room for immediate attention. New guidelines went out that we were to leave all patients with a score of 7 or below at home. (It subsequently changed back to level 5.) We left several houses knowing we had left that person to die. I had to pull over twice because my young, newly qualified colleague was beside herself. Weeping inconsolably. That is not what we do. We save lives. Many of our crew are young – in their 20s. Another shift it was another colleague, a young guy – distraught. It is the moral injury that we have sustained that will get us in the end, not the Covid. How do we live with that?

Did we get any help? Management introduced a tea truck that sometimes visited the hospitals. If it came round when we were there, we got a cup of tea and a biscuit! When I went off sick for three months with Covid, I fell through the cracks. No one contacted me at any point to see if I was okay. Full-time colleagues were much better looked after, but even so, we are a health service after all, and we don't seem to look after our own very well.

On the flip side, we were lucky. We carried on as normal. We still had a job. We met people every day. We went into houses where the person had not seen a soul for three weeks.

I did not tell my family all the things I saw in the early days when it was at its worst. I had to protect them. And it hasn't finished yet.

Above and beyond
ICU doctor

It is hard to reassure people when you don't know if they will get better or not. When so little is known. I remember a man in his 50s. He was so frightened. I found that hard. I found it easier to treat patients when they were intubated, even though it is a bit more impersonal. I think the nurses had the worst time on ICU. They know more than a lot of the doctors. They are so skilled and they usually work one to one. They had up to eight patients and teams of nurses with no experience of this specialised care. They had to stay on the ward the whole time in full PPE. We doctors go off the ward, consult, have breaks out of PPE. I was lucky to be in a big central London hospital. It never was chaotic, just very hard work that had often to be done at speed, and our senior staff were very supportive. Other hospitals were really struggling.

I am really inspired by all the cross-centre working, the international co-operation. Consultants working flat out here and in Italy, still finding time to compare notes, share findings. Loads of clinical trials. Really impressive. People do go above and beyond.

Celebrating Pride
Amy Hodkin, CAMHS clinical nurse specialist

As a frontline worker and a nurse in the NHS, the news of a new virus breaking out made me very fearful. I was working on an inpatient mental health ward for children and young people at the time. From an infection control perspective, this changed the entire way we were working. It meant we could no longer show how much we cared in our facial expressions, due to wearing masks, and we had to adapt to new ways of working. I was fearful for the young people, sad that they couldn't go on home leave, go off of the ward into the real world and have visits from family and friends, and worried about the effect of this on their recovery.

I had to instil a sense of confidence in my colleagues that, when they were on shift, I would keep them and the patients safe. The other element to this was my daughter, who was 46. I had to make an extremely hard decision for her to go and stay with my mum for three months until I could reassess the situation. I didn't want to put her or any of my family members at risk. So I was caring for other people's children and not being there for my own. I would sometimes sit in the car and cry before going onto the ward, I was missing her so much.

In the midst of lockdown, we arranged a Pride Party on the ward. I made invites that we gave out and we ordered wrist bands, flags and rainbow accessories for all the young people to have their own (while keeping to infection control policy and procedures). I felt that Pride was such an important thing to the young people on the ward and their identity, knowing that there was no judgement and that they could be themselves. I brought in a speaker, took song requests and my heart filled knowing that, despite everything they had to contend with, the young people got to do something with peers and staff who embraced them for who they are. Covid didn't put a stop to that.

It felt so precious
Pharmacist

I work in general practice and was in the team responsible for the vaccine roll-out for our local population. We were one of the first to sign up to do it. Then we waited for quite a while. Nothing. Nothing. Nothing. Suddenly, in early December 2020, all systems go. Find a place to do it, find refrigeration, make it safe to deliver 1000 vaccines a week. Then came the reports of anaphylactic reactions. The day before, I wondered if we were doing the right thing. We all felt pretty twitchy. No chance of learning from anyone else because we were one of the first. Then the vaccine arrived and I thought, 'Oh my God, we are really going to do this.' We carried it like a new-born baby, keeping it flat. It felt so precious. We started with the oldest but that meant it was really slow moving everyone around and we quickly ran out of disabled parking. Teething problems. Everybody was so grateful. It felt like a magical day. We didn't waste a single drop. We stayed on late to deliver them. All the centres did that. And if we had any left, we rang round to get care home staff down and clinicians. The people on the frontline. We were scrupulously fair. Those care home staff were really brave, you know. Real heroes. It is not talked about enough. One Saturday afternoon, we heard Covid had broken out in a local care home. We went down there, packed all the stuff in the car and put on full PPE and did the injections there.

Another pharmacist came see our operation so he could roll it out elsewhere. I rang him to see how he had got on back in his area. He said to me, 'That was probably the proudest day of my career.' He had been working as a pharmacist for 30–40 years and he retired soon after. I felt the same. Proud but nervous at first. So many people volunteered to help. The people who came forward early on to help us were incredible too. Retired doctors and an A&E nurse still working on shift at the hospital came and put in extra hours. Then the hospital doctors said, 'Why haven't you asked us for help?' Down they came – eminent doctors, Harley Street doctors – all stepping up. That happened everywhere. Then all the people doing the questions, queue-managing and in the car park. Fantastic. Really fantastic. We were pretty worried about the booster campaign. Thought we would be overwhelmed with requests. Instead, all the calls coming in were offering help. And the guidance kept changing. Phew! But really it was a good news story, and in the end really fun. Mind you, I was glad when it came to an end.

Grace and dignity

Jacqui Alexander, funeral celebrant

Being the celebrant at a funeral service is a huge privilege. Families trust us to hold space for them on one of the most difficult days of their lives. They tell us their stories and they open up their hearts to us as if we've known them for years. During the Covid-19 pandemic, funerals moved to a whole new level of hard. Funeral workers were the unsung heroes with key worker status. Every day, we heard heartbreaking stories. Every day, we apologised for the shortcomings in what we could do because of government restrictions. Every day, we turned up to do our best, even when the crematoria took away the hymn books and stopped people singing, and when they took away a family's right to have the curtains left open so they could glimpse the coffin for just one more minute or two. The funeral companies took away the limousines, took away a family's ability to carry their loved one on their final journey, took away donation boxes, took away a chance to see their loved one for one last time with a viewing at the funeral home, and the government took away the wakes and the gatherings afterwards.

The amazing families we worked with stood tall. They understood. Even when numbers of mourners were dropped to single figures and large families were left to watch the funeral of their cherished grandma online, their grace and dignity were outstanding. As professionals, we kept our distance, setting an example by hand-sanitising on the way in and on the way out, politely declining to shake the hands that were thrust towards us by those who were moved by our words, offering an elbow tap instead. Perhaps we looked uncaring in not offering a shoulder to those in tears, but that is far from the truth. We needed to keep safe for the overwhelming number of funeral services to follow. That didn't stop us, though, from giving a cheery wave of farewell, getting in our cars, and sobbing our hearts out.

Not ashamed of my sadness

Hasina Zaman, London funeral director

It was overwhelming in the first pandemic. I decided to stay open out of instinct. My father said. 'You need to keep going. You are offering a service people need.' There was so much we didn't know. Will I get the disease? Will my staff? Is it dangerous to do our job? And because two local Muslim funeral directors were not available, it became mayhem. I was working very long hours and I was worrying about my family. There are nine in our household. It was impossible to keep social distance there. Would I bring it home with me? My children were worried about me.

I like to do things slowly, offer real care and compassion, and it was almost impossible with so many deaths. The person had to be brought to us and kept in the body bag. It felt so wrong. When we went to the hospital mortuary, the staff were all in full PPE with bodysuits, but I could not wear it. It looked so awful. Like the terror squad. I only wore a mask. I kept washing my clothes at the end of each day and hoping for the best.

Our usual practices were not possible. Families could not care for the body at home, wash it and put it in the shroud. For a long time there was no viewing even. No prayers spoken over the person who had died. No chance to come and pay your respects and make peace with the person. No gathering in the Mosque. Only six allowed at the cemetery. In our community and in the West Indian community, it is expected that everyone will come to the funeral. The whole community is there. The Imams taught us that, in a pandemic, it was allowed to waive all these practices, but for families it still felt traumatic. And in the midst of all the rush, I was always trying to slow things down so people were really present to what was happening. A moment is still a moment if you are aware of it.

It all felt so strange. My walk to work felt so desolate. No one about. Like I had stepped into some weird apocalyptic movie. It was spooky and it all happened so fast. One woman said to me she could not come to see her husband because she was frightened for herself and her four children. Imagine having to make such a choice. Hard to find any peace with which to wish the soul on its way and ease its passage. Instead, lots of pressure and rules. Don't do this. Don't do that. There was so much fear about and that I think is very bad for all of us. I am lucky; I have a wise elder in my father, and he is always there for me. He said, 'Just remember what you are doing is for the greater good,' and that kept me centred on what was important.

One time, the registrar rang me at 7am in the morning and I just burst into tears. And I went on crying most of that day. My staff thought I should go home but I said, 'No, I am not ashamed of my sadness. I am not going to hide away.' So I told people when they rang that I might cry. I think that is important. I was grieving.

We were scared
Lucy Coulbert, Oxford funeral director

Right at the beginning of Covid, everything felt like a mad scramble. I remember watching the news coming out of Italy in particular, and just knowing this was going to be bad. In February 2019, I spent close to £15,000 on masks, body bags, gloves, aprons and full Tyvek suits. It seemed like a lot of people were just not taking it all seriously enough. At the beginning of March, I also made the decision that all of my staff would be wearing masks at funeral services. This was before any government mandate or law. I also had a big meeting with my staff and asked them all if they were still comfortable working with me. I told them I would do everything I could to keep them safe and would provide them all with PPE, which I expected them to wear.

I split everyone into teams and they all worked from home. Only I and one member of staff came to my office, knowing that we had isolated staff from each other so, if we got sick, we had healthy people to take over from us so our service to our clients wasn't interrupted. I really struggled for days with closing the office before I made up my mind. I know a lot of funeral directors didn't close. Kept their family rooms available and all throughout Covid. I just couldn't do it, though. I felt I needed to do everything I could to keep everyone safe, rather than follow what other companies were or weren't doing. Some companies weren't even giving their staff masks until they were made compulsory by hospital mortuaries.

The most difficult decision of all was we didn't allow anyone to come and see their person. While it isn't a terribly common thing for our clients to ask for, for some people, this was very difficult. We made sure we told everyone about this before they engaged our services. Even if they were okay with this, it was particularly difficult to explain it to extended family members and in the case of fractured families.

We were scared. The almost desolate roads. The horror of what we were seeing in hospital mortuaries. The utter rage some people had and directed at us. I know they weren't really angry at us, but we took the full force of people's anger and, at times, it became very difficult for us to cope with it. And I will forever remember the quiet fortitude of clients in accepting what I couldn't change because it was law and not my rules. Their gratitude for being allowed a funeral service at all.

At one remove
Joy Elliott, hospice counsellor

Sally and her husband had lived with his illness for four years. They had continued to enjoy their time abroad now that they were both retired. Covid then hit in March 2020, and they found themselves shielding, due to Jim's vulnerability. They still enjoyed their time in the garden and lived what Sally now realised was a very limited life, which was to be the last few months of Jim's life.

The change started in the August; not being able to accompany Jim to his appointments caused Sally much distress. She felt that she was not as connected to what was happening to Jim and found herself becoming more and more anxious. Services that had been face-to-face were now by phone, and this left her feeling very isolated.

Unfortunately, by the end of October, Jim was becoming more and more unwell. He was eventually taken to hospital with sepsis. Sally was allowed in to sit with him as he was very ill. On the third day, the staff in the hospital changed and a new member of staff requested that Sally sit two metres away from her husband. Sally found this very difficult, and having to hold her husband's hand through a rubber glove while wearing a mask has had a lasting impact.

Eventually it was decided that Jim would be moved to the local hospice. Jim was there for eight days before he died. Only Sally and her immediate family were able to be with him. His elderly mother, brother and sister had to make do with a video call – an added dynamic to their grief.

Having to isolate and not being able to make contact with friends had a huge effect on Sally's grief. The natural part of grief where you start to emerge back out into the world has been much delayed for her and others bereaved through the pandemic. Joining an online bereavement group and meeting up with four other ladies who were also grieving the loss of a partner allowed Sally to share her grief.

Eventually the bereavement group was able to meet face to face and find a space to acknowledge each other's grief and the struggles that they all had to deal with through the pandemic.

How was your lockdown?
Julia Samuel, psychotherapist

I am regularly asked this: 'How was your lockdown?' My brief answer is 'busy'. I did not make sourdough or learn to play an instrument; I worked. Harder than I have ever worked before.

In the years since I trained to be a therapist, I have come to recognise that I chose this work because I wanted to give what I most wanted to receive, and because being in meaningful relationship is profoundly important to me. The roots of this were certainly in my childhood and, of course, in human nature: we are hard-wired to relate and connect. The reason I tell you this is because the pandemic turned the volume up on all those responses.

It is why I volunteered to support an NHS team of medical staff working in an intensive care unit. I facilitated two lunchtime slots of an hour, every week. I was one side of the Zoom call, and the ICU team were in the staffroom, talking to me through a phone, taking it in turns to express the full gambit of emotion that you can imagine someone would feel in that situation. For confidentiality reasons, I can only tell you about my experience.

It was intense. My journal reminds me of some of my process: 'I always feel bad that somehow I can't offer enough, but I was glad they talked... so touched by the care they give patients'; 'I was proud today, excellent session... they were emotionally honest, and it felt an important part of keeping the team together... we discussed some useful coping strategies'; 'A painful session, I was tense, worried that we all felt worse afterwards!' There were nights I woke with anxiety from difficult images and stories; there were wonderful moments of black humour, of raucous laughter that sparked warmth and connection – a defence yes, but also a healthy protection in the face of the difficulties.

The pandemic had thrown us all into an alien and frightening landscape of grief. We were all in the helping profession, we wanted to make a difference and in our own way had to recognise the limits of what we could offer, accept that simply being present is of value. I could offer the curative power of listening, witnessing, being alongside someone, heartfelt care – although working with many people was more of a psychological juggle, and the work was therapeutic rather than therapy.

It was my job to hold steady, listen, be an empathic presence who named the team's process as they explored their individual difficulties, expressed their feelings and gained insight, and, through the collective sharing, normalised what they felt. I aimed to communicate that they weren't failing by being distressed; that they should not conflate their feeling with fact; that they may have felt they'd failed if someone died, but that did not make it so, and to encourage them to hold the messages from their head and heart side by side – sit with the discomfort of feeling guilty while knowing they weren't actually guilty.

Sometimes what was needed was practical – demonstrations of breathing exercises, suggested walks in nature. It was turbulent, with mis-steps from me, but overall I think it did what was needed: it offered emotional support to the individuals in the team so they could manage their own responses to the work, which in turn built resilience in the whole team to care for their desperately sick and dying patients.

The suffering of these individuals, and of many thousands of others, was invisible, locked away in our minds and homes – the mental health pandemic running beneath the health pandemic. The fallout has not been reckoned with and I have no doubt it will inform the content of our therapy rooms for years to come.

I was keeping people safe

Andy Paine, bus cleaner

At first, I was furloughed. That was hard because I had to live on £120 a week. I managed to get some gardening and window-cleaning work and I did get a lot of rest. I survived. I remember thinking that actually I could manage with less money and that I felt better in myself. A bit stronger. Living more meditatively.

Then they needed us back. Me and three others had to clean the interiors of the buses by hand with bleach. 30 buses a night. It took all night. You got quicker once you got the hang of it. We didn't get any protective clothing. You could wear a mask, but it was so stuffy in there I didn't want to. There were latex gloves. Then we got the fogger. It's a sanitising tool. It pumps out smoke and detergent and does a bus in about 30 seconds. It was just me using it. And noise like that triggers my voices. I am a paranoid schizophrenic. I'm used to the voices, to their nonsense, but the heat and sunlight triggered side effects from my medication. I felt rough. No help. The rest of the team outside and me inside. Then I brushed the inside, picking up all the rubbish, lots of discarded masks. Amazing I didn't get Covid. I did feel I was doing something useful. Keeping people safe.

You just had to take it

Irfan, delivery driver

The job changed with Covid in various ways. No more signing at the door, just taking photos and showing that things had been delivered. Masks all the time. Most people were so happy to see us. They were stuck at home. I was delivering games and other stuff they could do. A few people, usually old, were very scared. I understand that. I was worried about my mum – she's in her 70s. Some people, maybe two per cent, could be harsh and nasty. One time I was trying to deliver a bunch of flowers, but they just kept shouting 'Stay away! What are you doing here?' You just had to take it. Some people left out signs warning they had Covid and other stuff.

The workload went up. Usually we have one minute to make our drops to businesses and homes, but it went up to one minute 30 seconds because we had to spray door handles and all that stuff. I was working three more hours a day and there was no extra pay for it. The masks we were given were not much good. I started buying my own because I have a few contacts in China. I got through 1000 of them and then needed 200 more. They cost me £1 a day. But I needed to be careful for my family. That was who I worried about. Before Covid, I used to come home and have a cup of tea with them all but now the routine was get in, take off all my clothes, shower, do a test and then, once I knew I was clear, sit down with my family.

After the rules had changed and we no longer had to wear a mask, I still got shouted at. One woman was really nasty to me in a supermarket about not having a mask on. I said, 'The rules have changed.' She wouldn't listen. I took it on the chin.

Why did it take a pandemic?
Claire Stagg, rough sleeper initiative co-ordinator

I worked in a day centre for homeless vulnerable adults, seeing 40 to 100 people per day. When a colleague said he was worried he might not be able to go to Tenerife at the end of May, I said, 'Don't be mad, it will all be over by then.' Before long, there were scenes outside the centre of angry, distressed people as we managed numbers coming in according to Covid guidelines. Many people who live chaotically do not always have English as their first language. Trying to assess them was a real challenge. Clients frustrated. Staff frightened. We felt at risk. Some staff bailed out; others rose to the challenge.

Our clients were not scared. They live on the line daily. For many, their day is graft, score, use and repeat. What hit them was so many places being shut and begging being much harder as no one was about. The surprise was that cases did not skyrocket in the community, that no one was dying. We were amazed. Then we realised that our people tend to live isolated lives. Workers going to hotels turned into temporary hostels as part of the 'Everyone in' campaign found scenes of chaos. It's like Beirut, one said. A lack of understanding from management of our day-to-day challenges. Always being asked for numbers when we knew they could never be reliable. The number of rough sleepers is constantly in flux.

With the pandemic escalating at a furious pace, motivation was fuelled by some incredible changes. Teams and providers pooled resources and worked together to support clients and colleagues. We created a daily outreach team consisting of a homeless health care worker, homeless vulnerable adult support worker and local authority street homeless prevention worker. This dynamic team could assess and make decisions on the pavement. Symptoms, housing, substance support, food. A daily housing panel was created to identify vacancies and homeless referrals, to use all accommodation immediately. This joining of forces reduced multiple barriers. I was so proud of my team. We all know working together creates better outcomes, but ego, control and power prevents this. Covid forced us to drop these negative emotions, but why did it take a pandemic?

It took its toll
Social worker

This is the first time I have spoken about any of this. It went on for two years nearly. The impact has been huge on me, personally and professionally. There was a clash between my personal ethics, my professional boundaries and what I was being told to do. There was a very good care home in my district that lost 50% of its residents early on. We were told not to speak about it, not to let the press hear about it, not to warn the families of fellow residents. Some of my colleagues had relatives in there. Terrible. The bodies were taken out at night so no one saw the scale of what was happening. But the staff in the home were having to cope. Some of them decided to sleep at work because they were worried about taking Covid back to their families. Fear. It was everywhere.

No one knew what to do in the beginning. First of all, we were still making visits when we shouldn't have. We had no PPE, and then really poor-quality stuff. Gloves that didn't fit. All that. We got conflicting advice. Government would say one thing, the local authority would amend it, our managers would have their own take. We were like headless chickens, and it all moved so fast. I was surprised how we all reacted. People I thought would crumple weathered it out. Others I imagined being very resilient just collapsed. So then some of us had to stay on and stick it out, take on more caseload. Colleagues died. Service users died. And I have to say I could not join in with all that clapping on the doorstep. Not because I don't think the health workers were amazing. They were. But we were on the frontline too and it felt like nobody noticed or realised how tough it was for social workers and many others.

We were all exhausted. I asked for supervision to help me cope. I didn't get it. 'We just have to do our best and do our duty,' I was told. Then I would be told not to visit service users but to do assessments remotely. Imagine trying to do a video assessment with someone with dementia. They would have a carer with them but it didn't help. 'Who's that?' they would say. They didn't know anything about mobiles and tablets. They got distressed. I had to go against the advice and get in to see them to be able to do my job. In the end it took its toll on me and I ended up off sick myself for five months. I just stayed at home. I couldn't go out. Everything was going round and round in my mind about work. And I love my job. I love it. But I couldn't do it properly.

Left in the lurch
Police officer

Covid changed everything. I've never known so few calls for service as during the first lockdown. No bars and pubs for people to drink in and way fewer burglaries because everyone was staying home. However, management was terrified of being liable for someone contracting Covid in custody. We had to wear masks, goggles and aprons when bringing people in, and continued to do so even after medical staff had stopped wearing aprons in A&E. Half the time we couldn't even see properly as the goggles were misted up. But in the early days the attitude towards it was quite lax. I am now certain I first got Covid during a house search in March 2020, but no one was being tested at the time. I later found out that the homeowner was infected, but they didn't tell us and multiple people on different teams fell unwell.

Some bosses were slow to let people work from home, leaving some offices unnecessarily overcrowded. It was tricky at the start because many of the people who self-isolated due to a 'cough' were already regarded as work shy. I would also have felt bad isolating as it would have left my colleagues in the lurch and I didn't want to seem lazy. I was aware that a lot of my colleagues and friends were pretty complacent as we weren't worried about getting it. I am in my late 20s and I guess we felt a bit invincible.

We really didn't know what was coming

John Pearce, social services manager

Message from the Director of Public Health on 02/02/2020:

> The Government and NHS are extremely well prepared to deal with Covid-19. All necessary measures are in place to respond to any cases and to protect the public as the situation evolves. Please be assured that colleagues across the system are working tirelessly to address the ongoing situation.

Just before the national lockdown came into effect, in March 2020, I was working in the local social services, supporting frontline staff and the private care companies delivering care in care homes and in people's own homes. Cases of Covid-19 had begun to increase, but none of us truly realised yet the scale and seriousness of what was coming. Within days we were having increasingly desperate calls from providers not able to access the basic protective equipment to ensure carers' safety.

This composite email has been put together to illustrate some common issues.

> I am emailing you to inform you that the Home Care Agency have refused to continue visiting Mr H to provide care for him. He receives four calls a day, 30-minute visits to support with getting up, washing and dressing, support with food preparation and medication. Mr H is then supported to go to bed in the evening – another 30 minute call.

> During the visit from carer today, it was noted how Mr H had a high temperature and struggled to get out of bed without the support from two people (son helped carer). Mr H's temperature was 38 degrees Celsius. The carer called the paramedic who advised that Mr H and his son self-isolate for 14 days. Due to this, Home Care Agency informed me that no carers would be going into visit Mr H for the next 14 days. They will contact Mr H on the 14th day and review if safe to visit. Home Care Agency said they were following the government guidance.

Son has agreed that he can support with food and medication, although he is unable to give personal care. The minimal care support needed is 30 minutes AM and 30 minutes PM calls, whilst son is needing to self-isolate.

Please advise – they will need support from tonight.

Suddenly the military are on my email list; mortuaries and undertakers are asking me for body bags; staff are asking for reassurance on what type of masks to wear. We have gel but no bottles convenient to use. A local distillery helps out. I have new staff I've never met now working across the region trying to find the latest regulations and what they mean. We were all working crazy hours and beginning to feel the effects. The sheer pace of change was extraordinary. On occasion, the critical safety guidance changed twice in one day. There was a feeling of panic.

There were images on TV of medical consultants and nursing assistants gearing up in full hazmat suits and testing patients in their cars outside the hospitals. No images of what I was hearing about in the care homes. I was in contact with the public health outbreak containment consultant continuously, as the deluge of outbreak reports flooded in.

I had a call one night when Public Health England announced that, following an outbreak, we were to close a care home with immediate effect. Forty residents and all 12 staff living on the premises had to isolate and were not permitted to complete the care duties. We had residents needing medication and ongoing care in an hour… and staff must be found to do this. Who could help? The care staff were amazing, stepping up, coming up with solutions, organising rotas, bringing staff in, and the ill and vulnerable were looked after. This type of call I will always remember as a mark of the times.

Care staff were so brave. They just got on with the job as they knew they had to (and wanted to) deliver the care that undoubtedly saved many people's lives.

It was like a tsunami

Heidi Kennedy, registered home care manager

I am immensely proud of the team of home-care staff that I work alongside and support every day. Covid has had a significant impact on the balance between personal and working lives for frontline staff that is almost incomprehensible when I think about it. It has been like a tsunami.

Caring for the elderly and vulnerable at home presented challenges prior to the pandemic such as underfunding, staff shortages and lack of recognition for the complex work that home care workers deliver on a day-to-day basis. Then suddenly we found ourselves caring for individuals without the back up of district nursing staff, as all 'non-essential' visits stopped, GPs would consult on the phone, relying on carers for assessments when they could not communicate with the patient. The occupational therapists were asking us for measurements for equipment, and family members who normally provided social contact were in lockdown in their own homes. We just got on with it.

In March 2020 my stepmother passed away suddenly to Covid. In April, my close work colleague lost her younger 58-year-old sister, a care home worker, to Covid – the news was delivered to her by WhatsApp. Times have changed beyond recognition. The ripple effect became the tsunami when my dear father-in-law died in June 2020; him being able to die at home was a relief to us. What we did not expect was the lack of available medications, the lack of emotional support to him and my mother-in-law and the dilemmas we faced attempting to provide care and support to them during a national lockdown.

We chose to be with him to ensure he could be at home because he would have been isolated in hospital or a hospice due to Covid and it was inconceivable to think he would not be with his wife and family. That decision meant that he had his last meal at home, he was surrounded by people he loved and died in his own home. People often say to me, 'I don't know how you do this job.' We know that sometimes we cannot change the journey, but we can and do make a difference for someone dying at home. Our family were all with my father-in-law in the house when he died. This is something I strongly believe in: families should have choices too; after all, they must live with the tsunami of grief and rebuild their lives once a loved one is lost.

My concern is that the family and friends of those who are dying have no choice and miss out on the journey that enables them to say 'goodbye' or 'I love you'. Being able to share in the final moments of life as an individual transitions to death is a privilege. A peaceful passing can and should be shared by those who can and choose to be there. Covid has removed so many choices and has changed the way we communicate and think about death and dying. The most precious times are those spent with family and friends and are even more precious in the final moments of life.

I had to do my best for the residents
Residential care worker

The majority of residents who had capacity would constantly talk about how they felt like giving up on life because they were not able to see their friends and family in person and having regular telephone/Skype conversations only made them more miserable and lonely. During my time working in the home, there were a lot of resignations, from management to care staff and housekeeping staff. This impacted us a lot as most of us took on a lot more extra hours and it impacted our health.

Most of the residents were affected because they were getting different carers from different agencies, who did not know the routines very well. And they could not always find enough staff. I really felt the pressure to take on extra shifts because we had so many staff members leaving. Although taking on extra shifts was a personal decision, I felt like I had to do my best for the residents. This really took a toll on me mentally and physically because at times I wasn't getting enough sleep and I neglected my diet as I found that it was quicker to just get takeaways most of the time than to cook my own food. I also felt I should not be mingling with people even after the restrictions were lifted because I felt I was more likely be carrying Covid from the home. It took a long time for me to settle back into a normal sleeping pattern, which made life difficult.

Once the visiting restrictions were lifted, the residents' moods changed a lot. They were more positive, and some families decided to take their parents out of the home and chose to give them care at home.

Most of my colleagues felt the same impact on their physical and mental health. In the end I left. Now I am providing home care. It is much less stressful only having to worry about one person. I can provide much better emotional support.

The mission now is to undo all the issues it's caused

James Bailey, secondary school teacher

One thing I definitely noticed was increased anxiety and loneliness; due to less face-to-face socialising and more hours spent on social media, they were massively exacerbated. Exam or attainment stress was worse than I've ever seen it – and these students weren't sitting public exams! Four of my eight year-13 students at some point contacted me in tears; they were anxious, they were lonely. These were inner-city Londoners cooped up in tiny flats, often with large families. They had no life outside of those four walls and school became everything. The pressure, mixed with so much uncertainty, became toxic. They had no release. No normal adolescent way of expressing their frustrations or desires.

And the same was true for teachers. Teaching became our lives. We were unable to live outside of our role. I became obsessed over the mental health of particularly my sixth formers, who I'm also a form tutor to. I'd become anxious that their mental health would spiral and their despair would become too much to cope with. That somehow I was solely responsible for their wellbeing and that their mental health was something I could solve. We are not trained mental health professionals. So my own and many of my colleagues' mental health declined. But most of us lived in lovely flats near green spaces, and the vast majority of us had family members and friends to redeem the low points.

The mission now is to undo all the issues it's caused – the attainment gap between high and low achievers, the social anxiety that is rife in so many young people.

People seem to think teachers are invincible

Alice Matthews, teacher

I teach year 8s in a secondary comprehensive school in West London. All last year there was no joy in school – no clubs and events. All that was taken away – just learning, learning, learning. A lot of the time, whole groups of the children were sent home because of a positive test, and with teachers and children in masks, so much expression was gone on both sides and hearing people was so much harder.

Second lockdown, we worked on the normal timetable, using an online platform. It was hard – you are talking into a black hole. You can't tell what they are doing. Kids could not have cameras on because of safeguarding. We have a very diverse school. One could be in a really lovely home and one not. We could use mikes but there were often mike issues and chat could be used abusively to send rude messages to other students and teachers, so we tended to avoid it. I would randomly select students to send pictures of the work they had done that day. It was so easy for them to ignore you.

When I was assistant head of year, we had a rota between the head of year and lower school, phoning the most at-risk students to see if they had what they needed to work. In the second week, I rang one child who told me, 'I am doing half my lessons because I am sharing mum's phone with my brother.' We did manage to organise some laptops for them, but lots of schools did not have any budget for this. I was so aware of others picking up on abuse issues and so grateful I did not have to deal with that. Issues come up in school all the time and usually I can remove myself – go and do things I enjoy – but I couldn't do that. It was hard to put work down.

We are so grateful to be back in school and the classroom. Teaching remotely is not the job I signed up for. I don't want to be behind a computer. People seem to think teachers are invincible. We weren't prioritised for anything. No priority for vaccinations, 200 kids through our classrooms every day. It was scary. I never felt I might get it but thought I might take it home, and I worried about other staff members who were older or had serious health problems.

Not much thanks or recognition

Supermarket worker

It has been madness to be honest. I used to work school hours. I pick the stuff off the shelves for the online shopping orders. When the schools closed, my hours had to be night-time because of my kid. I would leave the house at 1am, start at 2am and sometimes I didn't get home till 5pm. I spent most of my afternoons on the sofa, asleep, with my nine-year-old daughter online-learning and my partner working from home. I was back in bed at 6 or 7pm. The orders went mad. Everyone wanting to buy online. We were expected to work at a faster rate. It went from 15,000 items per day to 60,000 per day. That's four times faster. Before Covid, most of the orders were done during the day and then the next-day orders would be done at night. The two just joined up. There was no let up. It had to be done.

Everybody was scared and very, very tired. Nobody knew who had it – customers, staff. We were touching stuff that the van drivers had touched, the customers had touched, and night shift colleagues had touched. There was not enough sanitiser to sanitise everything. As soon as I got home, it was overalls off and in the wash. We were worried about our families.

We weren't properly looked after by our company. The online delivery room is just a very small department out the back of the supermarket. There were 40 to 50 of us in work at the same time. No masks required. They were eventually provided but still you were not made to wear them. No chance of social distancing. We are timed on our shopping. Measures were put in place so you could skip an aisle or wait for a customer to move on, but then you were penalised for being slow. We were given high-vis vests to wear saying 'Please give us distance'. But customers would still approach us, lean over, remove their masks to ask a question etc. They gave other customers a good wide berth. We could not say anything because then we would get into trouble for being rude. It was pressure. Extra pressure. And not much thanks or recognition for what we were doing. We had some customers saying, 'We think you are doing a great job'. But others would just complain about our big trollies.

It did feel like it took a long time for people to recognise what we were doing. If we hadn't worked, you would not have got your food.

Some people actually lied
Sonia Oliver, organic veg grower

It started in March 2020. We just got endless orders for our organic veg boxes. The number trebled from 60 to 180 boxes. We were flat out. It felt scary. Our business has always grown slowly. Overnight, I had all these customers I didn't know, and when we reached our limit and had to say no, they could be very abusive: 'Fuck you, I have three children to feed.' I was really shaken. How could she speak to me like that? It is not as though there was no food anywhere. They just didn't want to go to the shops. Vegetables grow slowly. We could not produce any more. We took up some of our grass paths to make more room, but the only thing that grows really fast is salad. And there is a limit to how much of that you can eat.

After that, we shut our website down for a while and only took new orders from NHS workers who could show ID. Some people actually lied about working for the NHS to try and get a box. Can you believe it? But mainly people were very grateful, and I felt it was the first time people really noticed the importance of food growers. We became elevated in people's eyes. My former grower has young children and they were able to go to school all the way through because he was treated as a frontline worker. A bit like Dig for Victory in the war.

Years ago, I was in Poland, volunteering and supporting Solidarność in 1980/81. Things were really tough there. My grandmother queued up every day for food. It reminded me a little of that. The desperation. That time near the beginning here when some shelves were a bit bare in the supermarkets and no one knew how long it would go on for. I think people started connecting more with the idea of the growing and the importance of that and the need to think about food security. Developing countries have always struggled with these issues while they export to us. Maybe it's our turn now.

We will do it better next time
Iulian Firea, trades union representative
I am a key worker in the food industry, and I fed my family with low wages and Thursday claps for almost two years. It was fun, but not much fun.

I am also a union representative, and this put me in the front line of the frontline, with physical contact with my members and colleagues (about 1,500) on a regular basis, with worries and fights with the company about how on earth can we make things right and safe for all these souls. And I discovered that the enemy was not the company but the people around. The fear, the financial restraints due to imposed long isolations, the thoughts for the families abroad, the struggle to balance the safety on one hand and the bread on the table on the other: 'If I am seen as being sick, I lose the weekly wages. If I don't stay home, I might get someone else sick.' I've been a buffer between tons of governmental regulations, union safety advice and guidance, companies' group decisions and the undecided workforce. Undecided if they want or need to wear a mask, and when they got the masks, saying they can't breathe; undecided if they want or need to wear a visor, and when they got the visors, saying that they can't see; undecided to stay home sick and eat leftovers due to a flawed and poor sick-pay agreement or to come to work.

I've seen colleagues crying in debt after long-term sick periods, and I've seen people laughing because they are having more time off to spend with their families. I've seen colleagues with poor clothes or shoes due to closed stores and I've seen online shops gaining billions at the same time.

I've seen us losing our humanity due to the lack of interaction, fear of catching anything from the ones around, and pulling the last toilet roll pack from the shelf while baring our teeth to the others. And all this because of a tiny virus speck, because 'the unexpected' came into our lives. It was hard, a burden, a struggle, an unknown, a fear factor, a fight, sometimes even a laugh when seeing how the Prime Minister was a perfect model during the pandemic.

However, the hardest part when you go in a rollercoaster is the first time. So, I think we got this. We'll be better next time. Because we are humans.

Commentary
Liz Rothschild

How do we define where the frontline was – is? I would include all work that is essential to maintaining a healthy society, that cannot be conducted from home and usually requires some interaction with the public. The stories included here are from many, but not all, of the key sectors you could define in this way.

It was notable that a large proportion of the storytellers in this book who chose to remain anonymous contributed to this chapter. (All the storytellers had the option to protect their identity.) When you read some of the content shared here, you can see why. Their stories are of botched policies and procedures, and of requirements to keep silent. As the social worker says (p.23), 'There was a clash between my personal ethics, my professional boundaries and what I was being told to do.'

Some of these stories could have gone in several of the other chapters. Issues concerning the disproportional impacts on people from black, Asian and ethnic minority groups among frontline workers (and elsewhere of course) became brutally apparent as the pandemic unfolded. Patrick Vernon's commentary to Chapter 2 says more on this. There can be no question that social factors had much to do with the very different impacts on white and black, Asian and minority ethnic people in the UK – numerous government and scientific reports confirm this (Qureshi et al., 2022). This of course includes socio-economic deprivation. As Arundhati Roy searingly wrote in an article in the *Financial Times* about the spread of Covid in India (Roy, 2020): 'We can be sure it will be dealt with, with all the prevailing prejudices of religion, caste and class completely in place.' So also in the UK.

It was interesting to me so see how the understanding about who was a key worker shifted over the months. Initially, only the hospital medical, nursing and other health care staff standing between us and the virus were given this status. Many succumbed themselves to the disease when so little was still known about it, everyone was working in a state of crisis, protective equipment was scarce and methods of treatment were often experimental. Some had not even completed their training before they found themselves facing the most challenging health crisis in decades. Their voices are here, speaking from a range of roles. We hear the personal fears they had to manage while reassuring patients – concerns for their own health and that of their families; concerns that were viscerally real because of their daily encounters with the disease. Their stories reveal the astonishing dedication and hard work on minimal pay that they poured in, day after day, while dealing with the burdens of hot and ill-fitting equipment, if they had it at all. Chilling accounts also include the way in which paramedics had to revise their approach to assessing patients. In *Moral Injury* (p.12) you see how isolating it could become, and how these workers felt forced to keep silent about what they were seeing: 'I did not tell my family all the things I saw in the early days when it was at its worst. I had to protect them.' A social worker says, 'This is the first time I have spoken about any of this' (p.23).

A theme that emerges clearly from these accounts is that those who are in caring professions are often very unused to creating strategies to care for themselves. Their training does not emphasise this and there is a feeling that they should be able to cope. The Shout helpline volunteer reports a caller saying, 'I'm meant to save people, but I don't know how to save myself' (p.9). There are frequent stories here of staff requests for support being refused by management. The stark choices imposed by limited resources, escalating case numbers and the sheer pressure of work and high levels of anxiety will undoubtedly have a long-term impact on workers across many key fields. Of course, in some places valuable attempts were made to provide regular support, as psychotherapist Julia Samuel explains so well (p.19).

Looking forward, however, should we be concerned that some measures taken to relieve pressure on frontline health and medical services are continuing? The switch to far more remote working in GP surgeries – telephone triaging and consultation – has become a permanent feature. It clearly served an essential purpose at the height of the pandemic. Now there is a danger that convenience and staff shortages will lead to these practices being permanently adopted, resulting in a remoter relationship between doctor and patient becoming the norm. I share doctor and writer Gavin Francis's concern about the impact this will have on the practice of truly compassionate medicine at the community level (Francis, 2021, p.129). I believe it requires a sustained relationship built up over time – a deeper, not more superficial connection.

Gradually, however, the definition of 'key worker' used on billboards and other official pronouncements broadened out beyond the health and medical sector to include care workers and others who invisibly continued to maintain essential public services. But there were yet others too, in the business and commercial sectors, who risked their lives to keep us all alive, often because they needed the work to survive themselves.

The sense of not being appreciated was vivid for some. As the social worker says, 'We were on the frontline too and it felt like nobody noticed or realised how tough it was for social workers and many others' (p.23). As a nurse commented to me: 'I can't believe that in fact claps seemed good enough for professionals who are overworked and underpaid.'

It took me a long time to track down a hospital cleaner who was prepared to share their story (p.11). She is one of the few storytellers I did not have direct contact with. She thanked repeatedly the person who interviewed her and was clearly amazed we felt her story was important. It felt crucial to me to highlight those people whose work is seldom recognised but who are utterly crucial to the public health and care systems. Then there is the bus cleaner whose invisible work, at a high cost to himself, helped keep public transport safer (p.21).

The exposure to risk in the care sector was very considerable, especially when patients were being discharged from hospital back into care homes without being tested for Covid. Staff were not provided with adequate equipment or training and were supporting highly vulnerable residents. Despite this, in many places, they made heroic efforts to keep residents in touch with distraught families under very difficult circumstances and, as we can see in the accounts here, many felt keenly the confused isolation in which their clients were often living and dying. The relative invisibility of this sector at the time is surely a reflection of how their work is generally regarded and financially rewarded. The account by John Pearce, a social services manager, struggling to keep the sector functioning, is a sobering read (p.25). I hope we at least learn to value such key roles more in future.

It is striking to me that the lovely set of commemorative stamps about Covid that were issued in 2022 feature four health professionals and a hospital cleaner, a lab technician, Captain Sir Tom Moore and a delivery driver. No care workers. Other countries have recognised a far wider range of workers in their commemorative stamps.

We read here, and in other chapters, about the risks faced by teaching staff – they were the third most impacted profession after health workers and care workers in terms of Covid infection and deaths. And what about all the delivery drivers who were risking infection (and at times greeted with abuse by terrified customers) yet were essential to ensuring essential supplies were maintained and also that we could maintain some semblance of an enjoyable life. Yet, as reported in the *Independent* in April 2020 (Wood, 2020), drivers were being expected to continue driving without access to washing facilities and toilets at the same time as their workload increased dramatically. Very little provision was made to keep their working conditions safe either, as Irfan's account here describes (p.21).

Another vital element in keeping society functioning were shopworkers in food retail outlets. We know the degree of desperation and even aggression displayed when some items began to disappear off the shelves. Check-out staff were having to try to control panic-buying. Shopworkers had to face customers with varying degrees of respect for social distancing and mask wearing until it became mandatory. They were also working in environments that were slow to put measures in place to keep them safer such as directional flows around shop floors and screens. The comment by the supermarket packer (p.30) that customers treated her with less regard that their fellow customers reveals deep-seated attitudes about who is worthy of care and attention. Iulian Firea's story (p.32) also reminds us how confusing it all was, with health and safety guidance changing constantly and those it was intended to protect complaining vociferously about the inconvenience. Hindsight invites us to think it was obvious what should have been done at the time. It wasn't.

Most of us live without giving much attention to the origin of our food or other supplies – until they suddenly disappear off the supermarket shelves. Organic veg grower Sonia Oliver's story (p.31) shows us how strongly people can react in these circumstances, but also offers a way forward. She advocates for locally grown food. Just as the pandemic has revealed we do not all have to travel to work, so interest has increased in sustainable food sources and, for those who can, being involved directly in growing food.

One sector that seldom if ever got a mention on the news is mine – the funeral industry. My suspicion is that there was no desire to foreground our work and remind the public about death and dying any more than was necessary. For a long time the government website offered no clear guidelines on funerals, while the restrictions on weddings were writ large for all to see. At the same time I was receiving calls from the military, working with local authorities, checking out the possibility of provision for mass graves at our burial ground. Even when guidance did appear, it took some time for it to filter down to ground level and there was often confusion about what was permissible, leading to difficult conversations with families. As is well described here, the funeral directors were left to cope with unknown levels of risk as initially there was no understanding about how transmissible the disease would be after death. Some decided to close until the situation became clearer. This left those remaining open under even more pressure, but they too, like healthcare workers, were impacted by not being able to offer their usual service. Hasina Zaman says (p.16), 'I like to do things slowly, offer real care and compassion and it was almost impossible with so many deaths.' Lucy Coulbert honestly admits it was hard to cope at times (p.17). 'We were scared. The almost desolate roads. The horror of what we were seeing in hospital mortuaries. The utter rage some people had and directed at us.'

And there were discoveries. Some outdated practices were rapidly abandoned. A small example among many – the 'green burial forms' used only to be available in hard copy. Suddenly, an emailed version became acceptable. People also broke their reserve about taking photographs or livestreaming funerals. When it was the only way to include more people, those living abroad or people too vulnerable to leave home, they saw the value of it. That attitude remains, enabling people who still would not be able to attend a funeral for a range of reasons to feel included and even, sometimes, contribute. Other such positive changes in practice are reported here from different professions and many describe a welcome reduction in red tape, the forging of closer relationships with professionals from other disciplines and other countries. There was more efficient team working and flexible, rapid responses to changing circumstances. These are lessons that many intend to try and carry forward for the greater good.

We need to be sure that we insist our government funds the training of enough staff in key areas and pays them adequately to prevent all our key workers from either choosing other work or emigrating. All too frequently, it was the less well paid who kept the wealthier safe and cared for. Tea and biscuits from a truck, if you are lucky, are no substitute for fair reward for essential work.

References

Francis, G. (2021). *Intensive care: A GP, a community and a pandemic.* Profile Books.

Qureshi, I, Gogoi, M, Al-Oraibi, A., Wobi, F., Pan, D., Martin, C.A. Chaloner, J., Woolf, K., Pareek, M. & Nellums, L.B. (2022). Intersectionality and the developing evidence-based policy. *The Lancet, 399*(10322), 355–356.

Roy, A. (2020, April 3). Arundhati Roy: 'The pandemic is a portal'. *Financial Times.* www.ft.com/content/10d8f5e8-74eb-11ea-95fe-fcd274e920ca

Wood, V. (2020, April 29). 'I wouldn't let an animal use the toilets that we've got to': Delivery drivers fear lack of protection as they work through coronavirus pandemic. *The Independent.* https://www.independent.co.uk/news/uk/home-news/coronavirus-delivery-driver-safety-protection-vcovid19-spread-transport-hygiene-toilets-waiting-rooms-a9448071.html

Liz Rothschild is a performer, writer, celebrant and founder of the award-winning Westmill Woodland Burial Ground on the Wiltshire/Oxfordshire border. She won the Good Funeral Awards for the promotion of a better understanding around death and dying and is passionate about death education, believing that everyone benefits from daring to look our mortality in the eye. Her festival, Kicking the Bucket, ran bi-annually in Oxford for several years and seeded other work around death and dying in the city. With her Full Circle production company, she tours her show *Outside the Box – A Live show about Death* and does readings from her first book (published by PCCS Books), also called *Outside the Box*. www.fullcircleproductions.org.uk; www.woodlandburialwestmill.co.uk

Resources

Books

Clarke, R. (2021). *Breathtaking*. Little, Brown.

Down, J. (2021). *Life support: Diary of an ICU doctor on the frontline of the Covid crisis*. Viking.

Francis, G. (2021). *Intensive care: A GP, a community and a pandemic*. Profile Books.

Francis, G. (2022). *Recovery: The lost art of convalescence*. Wellcome Collection.

Private Eye. (2021) *Dr. Hammond's Private Casebook*. Private Eye Productions.

Samuel, J. (2020). *This too shall pass: Stories of change, crisis and hopeful beginnings*. Penguin Life.

Van Der Kolk, B. (2014). *The body keeps the score: Mind, brain and body in the transformation of trauma*. Penguin.

Media reporting

Boseley, S. & Mohdin, A. (2020, July 27). Daughter urges inquiry into Covid-19 deaths of bus drivers in England: Call comes after report says earlier lockdown could have saved lives in London. *The Guardian*. www.theguardian.com/world/2020/jul/27/earlier-lockdown-could-have-saved-lives-of-london-bus-drivers-says-report-coronavirus

Kenyon, P., Deas, A. & Johnston, C. (2021, October 3). Occupational hazard: The bus drivers who died of Covid. *File on 4*. BBC Radio Four. www.bbc.co.uk/programmes/m001009z

Tiernan, L. (2021, October 1). BBC Radio 4 investigates the London bus drivers who died from COVID: 'I won't stop until I get answers'. *World Socialist Web Site (WSWS)*. www.wsws.org/en/articles/2021/10/01/bbcr-o01.html

Thomas, M. (2020). *Mark Thomas' lockdown check-ups.* Wellcome Collection. https://wellcomecollection.org/series/XwROKRQAAGwR-YMk

Thomas, M. (2021). Keywords. *The Mark Thomas podcast.* https://soundcloud.com/themarkthomaspodcast/keywords-episode-1

Organisations

For workers who are unionised, your best source of advice and support is your trade union. Other less-prominent workers' organisations and organisations concerned with specific occupational issues are also listed below.

ACAS. Support and advice on resolving work disputes. *www.acas.org.uk*

Citizens Advice. Offering advice on a wide range of issues from employment to housing, domestic issues and benefits. *www.citizensadvice.org.uk*

Cleaners United. An alliance of trade unions and community organisations building a national campaign to improve the working conditions of cleaners in the UK. *www.centreforprogressivechange.org/cleanersunitedenglish*

IPSE. A not for profit support organisation for self-employed workers. *www.ipse.co.uk*

Nurses United. Grassroots network of nurses supporting nurses, including Nurses of Colour Network. *www.nursesunited.org.uk/campaigns/nurses-of-colour-network*

Samaritans. 24/7 helpline for anyone who needs to talk to someone. Tel: 116 123. *www.samaritans.org*

Shout. 24-hour confidential textline offering support. Text 85258. *www.giveusashout.org/*

Video

Levine, P. (2014). *Nature's lessons in healing trauma: An introduction to somatic experiencing.* www.youtube.com/watch?v=nmJDkzDMllc

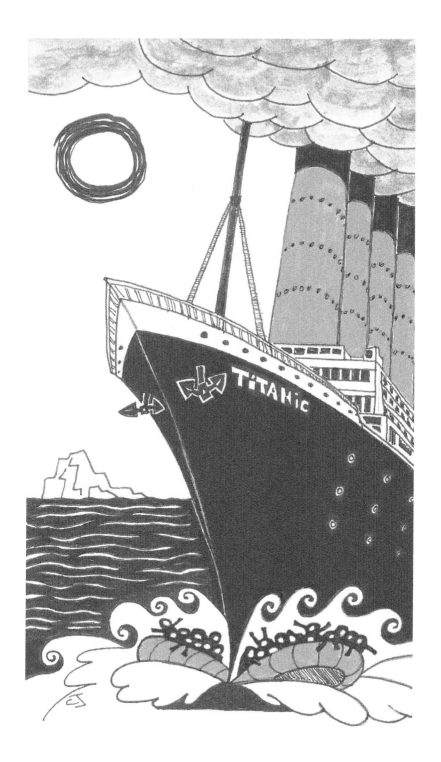

2.

We are not all in the same boat

'This is no time for cowards'

These words were spoken to rally colleagues by Dr Gamal Osman, a consultant in acute medicine. He knew his life was more at risk as a member of the black, Asian and minority ethnic community, and chose to continue serving his patients. He died in Bristol Royal Infirmary, where he worked. Many more gave their lives in service in many fields of work. May they not be forgotten, nor the lessons be left unlearnt.

Collective trauma

It was the first or second week of the first lockdown and my brother-in-law died. None of us really understood much about Covid-19 back then. It was all so new. My family wanted to gather to observe the usual rituals and to pay our respects. That is what we do in our culture. It is considered impossibly rude not to do so. My parents and parents-in-law found it really difficult to understand why we were saying they shouldn't attend any family gatherings. We found it difficult not to go ourselves. But we knew it was the law and we wanted to stick to the rules. Some of our family met just the same, and quite a number of them became ill.

My brother-in-law got very sick suddenly with acute chest pain, and when they called for an ambulance, they were told there were none available and if they thought he was really ill they would have to bring him in themselves. When they got to the hospital, none of them were allowed to stay with him. Luckily one of the younger members of the family knew someone who worked there, and they told them that someone needed to come in because he was dying, and we did manage to do that. It was brutal. In my family there were nine deaths. My cousin also had Covid, and he spent many months in intensive care. We were terrified we would lose him too, and his fight for survival became a symbol of hope among the heartbreaking losses.

This was before all the stuff came out about why the virus might be affecting Indian and Afro-Caribbean communities more. Before all the articles about black, indigenous, and other staff of colour being placed in more vulnerable positions, or people already having less good health due to economic injustice. We got the feeling we might be bringing it on ourselves. I got those messages from the media and from people I worked and studied with. And it is true that we live intergenerationally. We think that is important, and that makes it harder to isolate. None of the research on this stuff has been published yet.

Then, as the pandemic seemed to be easing here and restrictions eased, shocking stories started coming from India. There were multiple deaths. Stomach-churning numbers. People arriving at hospital and being told there was no oxygen and they must try to buy some or do without. Our community started raising money to send over medical supplies. I spoke to my dear uncle. He is a well-informed man, a professor of economics. He said to me, 'Oh dearest. This is India. People die in India. They die all the time of poverty and malaria. The world is only interested now because it is Covid.' People who had gone back had to be repatriated in a hurry. It was so frightening. There just isn't the infrastructure there to fight the disease.

As certain areas in England were put under tighter restriction, like Leicester, Manchester and Bradford, my community felt spotlighted. There was a feeling of accusation, and I began to wonder if people moved away from me in the tube because I was Indian. The Indian variant began to be talked about and I felt a heightened sense of risk and worried about seeing my family. We do feel less safe as a community compared with the rest of the UK population.

I am training as a therapist and what I see in my community is collective trauma. I am not grieving alone for the people I've lost; my whole family is grieving, my whole community. It has not even been consciously addressed yet. There has been no way to process the grief, and this is true of the wider population too.

We have been attending funerals online and feeling voyeuristic and not humanly in touch with the people we need to see and feel and know are there. When you are watching a computer screen, it is not a spiritual experience. Usually, the body would be returned home and considered a sacred object before the funeral rites, and then there would be 13 days of mourning. None of the physical rituals are possible, and when relatives are in care, it is taken even further out of our hands with autopsies and enquiries. We are a tightly knit community and we suffer a lot when we cannot connect at these times.

A community mourns

Yansie Rolston

Covid-19 was not on our radar. The hall at South Africa House was filled to capacity, with spill-over into the adjoining room as people – some famous faces from off the TV; others like me, just ordinary, everyday folk, with deep admiration – dressed up in our finery, gathered for one collective purpose, to wish Dame Jocelyn Barrow a happy 90th birthday.

We stand as she saunters in wearing a royal blue dress – a colour that describes the way many considered her – looking as vibrant and as fabulous as ever, beaming her trademark warm smile. Oh, what a night it was. We mixed and mingled, toasted and smiled, sang and clapped and at times welled up in response to the moving tributes.

Mainly we were preoccupied with reminiscing about the powerful inroads Dame JB achieved as a black woman coming from Trinidad and making the UK her home. None of us would know that the birthday party would also be her communal end-of-life ceremony, and I am grateful that I was privileged to be there. She passed on six months later, and gender, race, culture and Covid intersected as the community mourned.

Dame JB was no ordinary woman; she was revered by many for the ground-breaking role she played for black people. She was the first black governor of the BBC and also founded the Broadcasting Standards Council – no mean feat for a black woman, even in this present day. She was an activist, meeting with Martin Luther King Jnr and campaigning against racial injustice. She was involved in housing, leading on setting up the Community Housing Association, and in education she set up the Each One Teach One programme.

She was a pioneer and an inspiration. Dame JB was always sharing words of wisdom, offering help and support and giving oodles of advice. She gave the black community hope.

Ninth April 2020 – there was a frenzy of calls and texts – me asking them, them asking me, trying to verify the passing on of Dame JB. Nothing in the media – no media tribute to her remarkable achievements, not even from the BBC. The community mourned and it was in those moments that hope was replaced with reality – that the transitioning of someone as remarkable as Dame JB was met with media silence – an invisibility that is all too common for black women.

The pandemic reigned, so there was no celebration of her life, with the flair and flamboyance, pomp and pageantry that she rightly deserved. No cultural rituals of the wake and nine nights with calypso and steelpan music, off-tune singing, cards and dominoes playing, alcohol flowing and eating soup and West Indian food. Instead, the community she so powerfully impacted grieved alone. On the day of her funeral, it was just me, by myself in my living room, eyes leaking, with tissues in hand, watching CCTV footage of pews and a coffin, while listening to her grief-stricken family and a reverend pay their respects.

Almost two years after, the community still mourns!

Tipping point
Limor

Once, when I was travelling alone in Thailand, I made the decision to tuck myself away off the beaten path for a few days for Songkran – the Thai new year. I had been told that icy-cold water gets thrown all over anyone who ventures into busy streets during the festivities, and I thought the experience maybe wasn't for me. After 24 hours of rural isolation, I was stir-crazy and decided a new experience and a good soaking would be better. Given this stand-out memory of how I struggled to stay put for such a short time, I really expected that lockdown would be torture for me.

Covid lockdown was staying put in a different context, however. It was a privilege to be able to stay home and work remotely. Given the risks of mixing with others, being at home meant – for a time – a sense of safety in my isolation. I was coping – fearful of exposure to Covid, and afraid for vulnerable loved ones, but coping. I understood that the fear of disease and the challenges of isolation were shared, although not everyone had the privilege of staying at home, and for some, safety was contingent on being able to leave.

The media attention that followed the murder of George Floyd, however, evoked a second collective fear. As an ethnic minority woman in the UK, I have experienced and been disadvantaged by racism. I am, however, light skinned; people rarely place my background correctly as I look racially ambiguous, and I live and work in a context where I have some distance from the microaggressions and more overt acts that are daily experiences for some racialised people.

As a narrative researcher, I know and rely on the power of stories as vehicles to illustrate the differences in our lived experiences and as tools for evoking emotion. There was no escaping this particular story as it gathered power and was subsequently adopted into discourses that focused on different aspects. For me, it was a psychic threat – an example of how systems of power give licence to people in authority to enact violence at their discretion. My family heritage made this point all the more salient for me.

My social media feeds at the time showed that the story had similar effects on some people, but other versions of that narrative also emerged: 'If he was a criminal, the police were right to restrain him'; 'Now is not the time to protest…' The same people who had objections about protests and statues coming down didn't seem to have anything to say about the actual racism that was being protested. I wasn't the only one who noticed this; some of us had to withdraw from social media to preserve our wellbeing.

We knew early on that people of colour were disproportionately affected by Covid, but we didn't know why. People I knew, or thought I knew, were using their platforms to protest their right to freedom of movement and reject mandatory masks, while complaining about protests about the right to dignity and safety. I felt overloaded by the realisation that issues that were such a worry for some were dismissed as an inconvenience or an overreaction by others. When an expression of distress is met with silence, it has a silencing effect.

Whether the issue is vulnerability to a biological disease or a socially constructed one, there is a psychic violence experienced by people who are affected by issues that others can't empathise with. This goes for bereavement as well – those that feel uncomfortable talking about it simply don't. Another silence that resonates and isolates.

It had not been long since I had experienced the loss of a parent, but in the midst of this moment, my worst fears were realised, and I lost another. Everyone who had loved me through the entirety of my life was gone. I found myself at the intersection of multiple forms of grief. A metaphor often used to describe stress vulnerability is the bucket model – stressors are like water, filling you up until you overflow. We need to find ways to avoid reaching our limit, but when there are multiple sources flowing in, there's no shelter from the shock when the cold water hits.

Darkness descends on my eyes
Rahila Gupta, Southall Black Sisters

The door to the porch, which is stacked with shoes and slippers, newspapers and deflated footballs, hangs worryingly off one of its hinges when it is opened. Six people live in this small, decaying house. Sukhwant,[1] one of the residents, has been informed via WhatsApp that a caseworker from Southall Black Sisters (SBS) will be there soon with the week's grocery supplies and a subsistence payment of £50. She speaks with a small voice and every gesture she makes seems to diminish her presence in the world, rather than enlarge it.

She and her husband, Baljit,[1] live rent-free but barely tolerated in exchange for Sukhwant doing all the cooking and cleaning for the home-owners.

It has been weeks since both of them caught Covid but her body still aches and her back hurts badly. It doesn't help that she sits on the floor with her sewing machine, stitching for hours on end to make a little money on the side. She gets paid £8 to £10 for making a Punjabi suit, the traditional dress of her homeland – a tunic and bottoms held up with a cord. It takes her a whole day. She has no choice because neither she nor Baljit have the right stamp on their passports and so are not eligible for benefits and don't have the right to work, even though she has been in the UK since 2011 and he since 2004.

For the Covid self-isolation fortnight, they starved because she could no longer go to the Gurdwara for free meals. Her cough was so severe, she thought she would stop breathing.

---

1. These are not their real names.

Now, because of the tenacity of Covid, even that small income has withered away. For a while, with Covid's many stops and starts, there was a newly released pent-up demand for weddings. She had some business at last. But that soon stopped because people found that their incomes had been hit hard and they couldn't afford the frivolity of new clothes for weddings. If it hadn't been for SBS's intervention, the couple would have starved.

Sukhwant is wearing glasses. She says that she has been unable to do her sewing because 'darkness descends on my eyes'. She doesn't know whether it is the long-term effect of Covid or because she cries so hard.

She cries because, after five years of a relatively happy marriage, Baljit fell off a garage roof while working for an unlicensed building contractor and smashed his skull and ribs. He was taken by helicopter to a hospital in Oxford, where he had several operations and went into a coma for 12 days. She sold the little bit of gold jewellery she had to pay for her daily travel from Southall.

Although Baljit recovered physically, he became prone to terrible bouts of anger, which culminated one day in kicking her in the stomach and slapping her. When she told the doctor that his condition had worsened, he called the police, who put her in touch with SBS. But she didn't leave Baljit. She lives in hope that he will become the person he once was.

Finally, in May 2021, they got leave to remain and could claim Universal Credit and rent for slightly improved accommodation.

Further operations have calmed Baljit down, but his strange behaviour continues. He hangs his slippers on his ears, he switches the lights on and off, he mutters under his breath. His anger is unpredictable. She leaves the room and waits in the kitchen for his anger to subside. She hopes he will get better. Meanwhile she cries.

The bill they received for £1.7 million for Baljit's treatment from the NHS still hangs over them.

https://southallblacksisters.org.uk

The asylum seeker

Nawaf

I was an asylum seeker when I had to flee my country and moved to the UK in 2015. The pandemic has made the already difficult and long asylum process more horrific, which has had an immense detrimental effect on my mental health and that of all others who are in the same situation. Asylum seekers get £39 per week paid through a prepaid card. The card is not permitted for online purchasing. When I contracted Covid in 2021, I had to stay at home for two weeks as I was following the government guidance then. There were some days when I was left without food because I could not use my card online and couldn't leave the house, and sometimes I had to rely on local charities to deliver me some food.

However, there is nothing compared with losing a loved one. It was the most difficult time in my life and for the whole family when we lost my brother, who was in his early 30s, at the beginning of the pandemic, after he had contracted Covid. I was unable to be with my family not only because of the Covid restrictions but also because I was not allowed to travel abroad while I was waiting for my application to proceed in the UK.

With all that I went through in my life and in the past two years of the pandemic, there is always a light at the end of the tunnel. We are getting closer to the end of the pandemic and I finally have got my right-to-remain status decided in the UK. I am hopeful and optimistic about the days and years ahead.

Pandemic kindness

Yasotha

I am a Hampshire-based GP, but previously I worked as a doctor to the homeless. When we moved to going out onto the streets as part of our patient contact rather than using clinic rooms, things unseen were made visible. There were very few people on the streets during lockdowns; it was like a ghost city. Those who were on the streets could not be overlooked and were more able to behave naturally too. When restrictions were relaxed you would notice the difference ; you were always conscious of being overheard or that there might be people watching our more vulnerable clients, provoking hesitancy or even aggression during visits. As I started working more closely in interdisciplinary teams, I began to realise that our medical model is all about success being seen in terms of diagnoses and clinical plans, not the nuances of holistic practice and building a team around the individual. It is not inclusive and does not prioritise relational working that serves patient care around individuals belonging to minority groups. Self-help can be a load of trollop in relation to people who find themselves homeless. It's often advice that is pitched at people with good social capital and disposable income. Mantras like 'If it does not serve you, leave' or 'Change you' are just callous when reflecting on how intractable homelessness can be and the context around it. It also places far too much responsibility on the individual when, as a big society, we need to reflect on more external safeguards to protect us all from being at risk of finding ourselves in this situation.

During lockdown, there were a couple of parks we'd have to pass through in order to get to the city area, and the gulls, pigeons, ravens and squirrels seemed much happier but also quite a bit more hungry. The bins were unnaturally empty and the footfall of food debris and bird feeders was very low. There was a gentleman, one of our clients, who you'd see using his allowance to buy bird food or sharing what he was given to feed the park animals. It was the kindest thing I think I have seen in a really long time. These acts were not isolated either. Our clients' lives were not easy, and they could be forgiven for sparing no kindness to anyone or anything. I strongly believe, if they had better years when they were children and young adults, they could well have been flourishing within society and not struggling as much as we saw. Sadly, some will remain trapped in homelessness as some contexts are simply inescapable. The acts of kindness these individuals showered on creatures they could not get anything back from stands as an example to us all.

Food poverty

Steve Benham

When I finished work on the Underground about eight years ago, I went to help more regularly with the food bank in our local Methodist church, stacking stuff away, checking the sell-by dates, serving tea, chatting to people. My wife, Marie, cooks. We serve lunches and teas; there's advice from Citizen's Advice Bureau, we top up people's electric sticks. I'd have a laugh, maybe do a jigsaw or two. Some people tended to be unemployed or on zero-hours contracts; others were homeless. Some had issues with drugs or alcohol. They were people who were lonely and struggling to get along. Then came lockdown and no one came in. We did some deliveries or put the bags outside for them to take. The local cookery college donated the food they couldn't use. We started to see people we'd never seen before. The working poor. They may have been on the margins, or close to it, and the pandemic pushed them over the edge. Some couldn't manage on furlough or had been made redundant. And with some of our regulars, when they did finally come back, you could see how it had affected them. One lady is so much more reserved. We try to cheer the kids up. Give them a bit more chocolate even, though I know it's not really good for them. We get some very generous donations.

Marie Benham

While I am preparing lunch and cooking, I am serving coffee and teas. We do a regular day most weeks. The one thing I really remember about that time is I noticed the clients who were coming in were different. They had had jobs. One lady was a hairdresser who had had her own business and had a family and so on. She said, 'I never ever thought I would come to this,' and she was quite distraught, as you can imagine. She said, 'I have always looked after myself and I don't know what to do.' People were quite shellshocked. One young father came in and he was simply dazed. He sometimes wasn't quite listening to what you were saying. He couldn't believe he was there – it was sheer desperation. He had been on a temporary contract and suddenly found his job didn't exist anymore. He said to me, 'It's my wife's birthday. I've nothing to give her.' We have a box on one side for this and we sifted through to find something suitable.

The people I am used to seeing are families who come in the summer holidays when the free school meals stop. It transitioned. We had to go back to basics and explain how the food bank works and about their employment rights and where they could get help, what other avenues they could try. You could feel the fear. They thought they might be turned away. We never turn anyone away.

Covid behind bars

I had to do two more years in the open prison. The last of my 14-year sentence. This was 2020; I had a job lined up (you can work in an open prison), and then the epidemic hit, three months in. No visitors or home visits or town visits. You could use the phone, but it wasn't the same. People began to lose contact with their families.

There were outbreaks of Covid in the prison. It had to be the staff because they were coming in and out. Some of them refused to be tested. The PCR test took three days to come back. I guess they did not want their lives outside to be restricted.

I am in contact with people. People I know joined me a year later in the open prison. They brought terrible stories of lockdown 23 hours a day. Each landing at a time together for food (30 mins) and exercise (30 mins). They were very depressed and down. Really horrible. The guy I was friendly with from The Mount couldn't wait to get out of closed conditions due to the Covid. All on their own in single rooms, like being in solitary. Yeah, there's a TV with six or seven channels, a radio, but if you have noisy neighbours booming out the music, you can't go and find a quiet place anywhere. Like a torture chamber. No insulation. They were angry about lockdown. Saying it's not necessary. Why are they doing this to us? Felt both abandoned and under siege. Little hope of getting out of it because it went on and on. Not much sympathy from the staff. Self-harming is likely to have increased. You see people with like scars on their wrists – using a razor to try and feel better. People say you are lucky, you have three meals a day and you don't have to pay for it. They just don't know.

Layers of deprivation
Gordon Knott, Director, Croydon Drop-In

A 14-year-old person came to see us recently. We had met three years before, when she'd needed support with her selective mutism, which started when her family had been moved into the borough. She'd started at a new school and was being bullied about being eligible for free school meals and not having the money to be able to afford the trendiest brands of clothing and footwear. She was back to see us again following the death of her step-father, which led to her, her mother and her younger sister being moved into one-bedroom accommodation. During lockdown, Mum was expected to home-school the two girls, so we loaned the family two laptops to help with that, supplied them with vouchers for food banks, and our advice and rights advocate worked with the family to negotiate with the council for more appropriate housing and with the school to prevent the younger sister being excluded.

Pre-Covid we were already working with the impacts of ingrained discrimination, insecure housing, poverty and austerity, and since the pandemic began, we found the following issues emerging:

- Parts of the community living in poverty had limited access to the internet or struggled to find the money to top up mobile phones so that the offer of a helpline meant little to them because they couldn't afford to make a phone call in the first place.

- Parents/carers were asked to assist their children's home education when they might be a speaker of another language or when their own levels of numeracy and literacy were not proficient enough to assist their children.

- Families were locked down with other household members when schools and workplaces were largely closed, placing much pressure on relationships.

- Adults moved into unemployment or zero-hour contracts.

- Existing Universal Credit claimants saw the benefit reduced and were worried how the system would cope with one million-plus new applications.

The impact on the mental health of children and young people is still revealing itself. In particular, we are alert to the vulnerability of looked after children, LGBTQ+ young people, and cohorts of children and young people transitioning across primary, secondary and tertiary settings who have had their education disrupted. Young refugees and asylum seekers are being re-traumatised by the lockdowns as it reminds them of the time they were trafficked/confined/exploited. We are also seeing a rise in the number of young people who are coping with an increase in grandparent/parent/relative illnesses and bereavements, as well as a rise in domestic violence incidents.

When you overlay our map of service delivery with the map of community deprivation in the borough, the areas match exactly, and this is no coincidence. We intentionally target our services towards areas of high need as we know these communities are disproportionately disadvantaged. The number of children and young people who access free school meals is higher than the national average, and 16% of children live in low-income households. On average, five children in every classroom have a diagnosable mental health condition, while 75% of all mental health issues are established by the time someone is 18. However 75% of young people who are experiencing mental health issues aren't receiving support.

Never mind whether the glass is half full or half empty, as long as it remains refillable, then there is hope.

What if you got Covid and couldn't communicate your needs?
Katie Peacock

I care for a 57-year-old man who has a learning disability, autism and a physical disability that means he is unable to stand and so he gets about on his hands and knees indoors. John (it's not his real name) is clinically vulnerable. Outdoors, he uses a wheelchair, pushed by his supporters. For the past 15 years he has lived in his own bungalow, supported by his own small team of personal assistants who know him well. John sees the world in his own unique way and he has very strong preferences for how he wants his environment to look and feel and about the clothes he wears. If you didn't know him well, you could end up causing him to become extremely distressed. He does not accept most instructions unless they are sung to him, which immediately works.

When Covid first came on the scene, none of us really knew what to expect and we were actually pretty frightened. We were frightened in general about Covid and what it might do to any of us, but there was a greater fear of what would happen to John if anything happened to his team. What if he ended up in the hospital and wasn't allowed to have anyone accompanying him? We knew how disastrous this would be. He would become very distressed and all the old habits we had managed to resolve would return – biting himself and getting highly stressed. So we created a body map. A head-to-toe plan of what John needed to keep alive. We succeeded in getting all of this vital information onto one page and we put it together with a copy of his most recent benefits letter, his medication chart and a letter with a list of where to find other essential things in his home. We included codes to his iPad where he stores his favourite music and where to find his money etc. It was surprising how much of a relief it was to us when all this information was collated in a simple 'at a glance' format.

Despite our intensified hygiene routines using PPE, one of our team got Covid. John caught it from them and then I got it. Nothing for it but to stay with him, keep all other staff away and hope for the best. Very luckily, we were neither of us badly ill. It was 10 days until we both tested negative.

The whole two years was an incredibly worrying and uncertain time and brought home just how precarious John's situation could become if he suddenly found himself in an overstretched, busy hospital where staff simply did not have the experience or time to understand how to work with him.

Connections were lost forever
Liz

As the pandemic approached our world at Christmas 2019, we began to notice signs of dementia in Kenny, who also has Down's Syndrome. He loved family, walking along the canal, and coffee and cake in a café. His support team made sure he had a good life, and the local community always had a smile and a wave for him. Lockdown changed things. As we negotiated the new reality to keep him alive, we stopped him from living. Connections with people and places were broken, lost forever. Staying indoors (he loved to shake hands with everyone) brought health problems, vitamin D deficiency and loss of strength. He retreated into himself, grew sick in body and mind. Precious months and years were lost to isolation. As I write, I am sitting by his bedside as his life slips away.

Without breaking an egg
Pam Douglas

I work with young women in Gateshead aged 12–19 who are referred to us by social services, schools or mental health services, or self-refer. Many have poor mental health and low self-esteem, lack confidence and social skills and are at risk of exploitation. Some are pregnant. We aim to build their confidence and skills so they can reach their potential. When Covid happened, we decided we had to close the office, but we did not want to close down the service and go on furlough. Working online was better than nothing but did not work well for quite a number of our young women, due to lack of privacy, data, phones and so on.

In the first few weeks we delivered quite a few food parcels to families who would normally have had free school meals. The schools had not reacted quick enough to sort out any vouchers, so many families found themselves struggling to feed everyone. When we were doing this, we realised how important our visits were, not just for the food but because it meant we still had contact with the young women.

We were able to secure some extra money to allow us to put together 'care packages', which we then delivered to every young woman (and their siblings) every week until the end of August that year. One hundred packages a week. This enabled us to spend some time with them, sat outside on their doorstep. We took them pamper stuff, footballs, books, puzzles, a wonderful wooden box full of useful things to help them with anxiety, frisbees, art materials, soil and seeds to grow sunflowers (it was a wonderful spring), the ingredients to bake a cake, including two fresh eggs each, which we delivered without breaking any. Then we did an online baking session together... hilarious! We were also able to give out more practical things like mobile phones, laptops and SIM cards.

Some of the young women had their babies during lockdown and were very much alone. They didn't have contact with other young mums but we were able to support them, again by sitting on their doorstep and giving them time to talk and share how things were going.

A wonderful moment came in April 2021 after the third lockdown. Two young mums had been very careful and not seen anyone other than their family, so the babies had not seen another baby in the nine months they'd been in the world. The look of delight on their faces when the babies saw each other and reached out to touch each other brought a few tears.

The appreciation we had from the young women and their families was immense. They felt we had gone above and beyond, when most other support services had shut down or went to telephone only. The joy with which we were greeted each week was priceless.

This experience changed how we saw ourselves as a project and as workers. Our willingness to embrace change to meet the needs of the young women, to step out of our comfort zone, has improved not only our relationship with them but our working practice more broadly as well. It has shown us that we are not a project that just does the same thing year after year; we're a project that is adaptable and agile and can face whatever the future brings with renewed energy and confidence.

The right to choose

When the new Covid vaccine was first approved for mass roll-out, I carried out as much in-depth research as I could from the credible sources I could find. I read the Pfizer study papers, articles in trusted medical journals and other reliable sources of information in order to reach a reasoned decision on whether or not to have the inoculation. I finally decided there were too many unanswered questions and no apparent access to the essential answers, so I chose not to.

At the time many friends were asking each other if they had had their injection and I had no hesitation in saying I had decided not to do so. I could never have imagined the effect giving out that information would have on my life.

Over the following months the government employed behavioural scientists to 'nudge' the population into more and more altruistic reasons for being inoculated; it was no longer to keep *you* out of danger but for the sake of *others*.

At the same time, a campaign was developed against those who had chosen not to be inoculated. It was and remains centred around name-calling and public shaming. I feel like a conscientious objector and 'unclean' member of my own society. Longstanding friends and some close family members refuse to see me or be in any contact with me. Fortunately, I do have friends who, like me, have chosen not to have the injections and some who have had them but respect my personal choices.

In my wildest dreams, I would not have contemplated that our world could have come to this: family against family; friend against friend; neighbour against neighbour; majority against the individual. It is truly ugly – yet the saying 'The darkest hour is just before dawn' rings true for me.

'Clinically vulnerable'

In the complicated world of Covid, my part is a small one. Yet it has profoundly changed my life. I am nearing 60, and lockdowns and the long isolation periods have at times been enjoyable, at times lonely. Never boring.

Financially, my income has been halved or more. My home is under threat, a threat that changes with each month and how much I can work. My confidence in how much I can influence that has reduced.

Most critically, it has forced me to face up to a long-term health condition that previously I have 'hidden' from the majority of friends, family and, most critically, patients. I have chronic blood cancer.

Blood cancer has a vibe that people respond to. They don't hear the first word, 'chronic', or that I have been living with it for 20 years. They focus on it as an immediate threat. Indeed, that was how I was introduced to it myself when knowledge of the disease and how to manage it was limited. It is rare still, thankfully.

However Covid suddenly put me into a government-labelled group of clinically extremely vulnerable people. Many letters arrived addressed as such, and 'shielding' appeared.

Having never thought of myself as vulnerable, despite taking a daily chemotherapy drug, I only ever tried to avoid people with infections, but not obsessively so. My strategy had always been to carry on as normal as much as possible. The new label was an uncomfortable shock. The fact that I was 'shielding' was a clue that something else was afoot.

This forced me during the first lockdown to re-evaluate, be honest with myself and start explaining it to family and friends. I then, with support from colleagues, also took the step of starting to tell patients.

I am an acupuncturist working from home, running a full time clinic.

So I fall into the categories of:

- working from home (good)
- meeting members of the public (very bad)
- close contact for an hour with each person (very bad).

This picture is mitigated by PPE and screening, talking to each patient before arrival about what risks they may have been undertaking prior to the appointment, checking temperatures, and serious cleaning and airing of the room between sessions. To enable this to happen, I had to come clean as to why it was important we all took it seriously.

Luckily this process has gone very well, everyone has been supportive and responsible and there has been not too much dwelling on my actual health. Phew.

However, what nags at my fully vaccinated self, about to face a fourth vaccine, is I truly don't know the risk I run.

I don't know if Covid would give me a sore throat and a bit of a cough or if I would die.

It's that stark, and it's the risk I run daily in my job, or if I dare to enter a shop or (for me, more likely) a hospital clinic. It's a weird form of Russian roulette. Daily.

In reality, it would likely be serious and I would eat up scarce NHS resources, so I remain cautious. I also remain vigilant because, without my input, my elderly mum would suffer greatly, and that thought tortures me a little.

And a little bit of my optimistic self says maybe not... maybe it would be okay. But it's a risk I cannot take.

Stay at home, protect the NHS and save lives

23 March, 2020: Government advises us all to 'stay at home, protect the NHS and save lives'.

I'm 73, I have worked as a self-employed complementary health practitioner for 21 years. My work is one-to-one, including touch, so I had no choice but to close down my business.

The government immediately awarded generous furlough funding and business support to its employed citizens. Meantime, the self-employed waited... and waited... and waited in disbelief at the Chancellor's lack of acknowledgment of the plight of millions of people in the self-employed sector.

22 April, 2020: One month later, Chancellor Rishi Sunak revealed Covid-19 Self-Employment Income. The stipulations were rigorous, incongruous and confusing. I did not qualify for any support as my self-employed income had been slightly less than 50% of my total income during the previous three years. I have a state pension and a very small private pension, which together pay my rent, and I live on my self-employed income. I therefore had no visible means of surviving and no idea how long I would have to be without an income.

With some generous help from a friend and a family member, I lived very meagrely for a couple of months while I worked out a plan for keeping a roof over my head and affording some food to eat. I knew that food banks were an option but that is a humiliating contemplation for everyone. After a deep and fascinating dive into the fundamental principles behind my work, I created a new way of working with people online and managed to get a small amount of income coming in, and could provide some support for others who were struggling in many ways.

Many self-employed people were in more desperate situations than I was – I had no family to consider or young mouths to feed. The stories I read on the Facebook group 'Excluded UK' were heartbreaking – with not a few successful suicides reported.

I have never been truly traumatised in my life, but this was real-life terror. Being prevented from earning a living, having no idea how long the situation would continue and discovering I did not qualify for any financial support was like Alice in Nightmareland. To experience our government regarding millions of its hard-working, self-employed citizens as of lesser entitlement than those in paid employment was shocking.

I managed to get through and am now re-building my business, some of which remains online. It was not all in vain, as I learned many new skills and deeper understandings about the work I do and of my own resilience during adversity.

Left high and dry

Claire Bateman

I am a cleaner working in holiday lets. When Covid hit, I was working for several clients. One of them started buying a lot of new properties during lockdown and advertising them for NHS workers. This enabled them to claim money from the government to cover costs and ensure their maintenance teams got some income too. Some tenants were NHS workers wanting to keep their families safe, but a lot of the people who came were just wanting to get out of the cities or people who could not get back to the countries where they lived.

It didn't feel right to me, but I was told, if I wanted to keep working, I'd better keep my gob shut. I was told to tell anyone who asked that they were NHS workers. And all those grants the employer got did not help me. They treated it like their nest egg. They built a swimming pool and then a jacuzzi. Meanwhile, I was struggling to pay the bills and having to use a local food bank. They told me to apply for benefits. My trouble is that I don't qualify for any government help because of the number of hours I work. I have an autistic son and I cannot work full time. But we need that income. We have ended up £2000 in debt.

And I did not feel safe. There was no additional protection. I normally buy all my cleaning equipment, but under the Covid regs, hand sanitiser, mask packs and aprons should have been provided. I got nothing. I just had to do my best. I bought as much sanitiser as I could and masks. Then, when I had finished work, I would change in my car and put my clothes into a black plastic bag and wash them as soon as I got home. Sometimes I was changing in the snow. I survived, and actually none of us did get it, so I feel very lucky. Not everyone treated me badly. Another client kept paying me and always rang to check on me and found work for us to do so we never felt we were getting something for nothing. They helped us survive through Covid, but they only have one property.

We've been here before

Tomos Williams

When it first started, my hatches were pretty much battoned down already following three months in bed after intensive treatment for my throat cancer.

Three months of sleep and not much else, apart from A, who was always there and always loving. There weren't many days when I didn't cry, and when I did, his arms were always open and I was always held.

March 2020 and I started to think that maybe I could walk further than bed to chair and back again. Maybe I could even go for a coffee.

And then we locked down so, instead, I curled up in my armchair, under my blanket and thought 'Ha!' when I heard the complaints, 'Welcome to my world'. And I thought about...

* Flashback to the late 1980s* – I'm sitting in a pub. Four of us round the table. S has a new KS lesion on his neck. We don't look at it and we talk about other things – cruising and outfits and pop music and tequila slammers. I'm in lust with (a different) A and I'm struggling. I don't know who I am trying to become, what I should be doing, and I'm being told that, because I don't know, I'm likely to die of ignorance. I'm being told the people round this pub table, who – at least in my imagination – do know and have become who they should be, are

to be steered clear of. I'm desperate to be intimate, to be physical, to be sexual. I decide that I have to behave as if I have 'IT'. I'm told that what I'm seeing across the table is the tip of the iceberg. I hear that the things I haven't discovered yet have to be constrained. I'm told that I have to police my own desires and my contact with other people. Nobody talked of a pandemic then. People talked of a plague.

Fast forward to 2021 – We are here, just A and me. My A. We go for walks, we shop online for baked beans and coffee. We watch stuff and read stuff and make stuff. A does things in the garden that he's been meaning to do for a while. We wear masks and keep apart from everyone else.

For the second time in my life, I behave as if I am already infected. And, once again, I am policing myself and my contact with others.

Since then, restrictions have eased and re-tightened and eased again. Parents have got older, a grandchild has arrived. We've been on trains (always in masks, even when nobody else was) and gone into actual shops. We even had people round for food and sat inside. It felt weird.

It seems self-evident to me that we will be revealing the effects of all this for a long time. I have learnt that I'm unlikely ever not to be in recovery from cancer.

There is trauma; there has been, for so many, grief. There has been waste and incompetence. There has been selfishness and thoughtlessness on a scale I've never seen before.

But there has been gentleness too, and kindness. There have been flowers left on the doorstep and nourishing soup delivered. There have been the two metre smiles and 'thank you' when we step off the kerb. It is the nature of these things to be delicate and fragile, that they don't make the news. Questions are not asked in Parliament about generosity. But, just as, thanks to my illness, I have felt more blessed and have learned to trust more deeply the love I receive, I hope that, amongst the therapy and the recriminations and the re-ordering, we remember the little things.

Locked down and locked out (again)

Sarah Pickthall

The start of that first year of Covid, things were looking quite bright, despite drastic cuts in social care – things that disabled creatives and consultants like me were making the case for and winning through – access requirements to be met and arts to be more inclusive.

That rapidly changed as we went into lockdown and we again were portrayed in the media as helpless and unable to fend for ourselves, with 'vulnerable' pasted across our doors. That's not to say some of us weren't clinically vulnerable; we were, and we needed that recognition of that fact. But we were also really adept and adaptive, with an already honed and natural set of skills in orienteering an inaccessible world. It wasn't all doom and isolation. Living with chronic fatigue and pain, I relished staying at home, conserving my energy and being my best Zoom self. During those first six months, I moved all my work online, including my global leadership programme, Sync, which I used to travel extensively to deliver, and by using captions and sign language, we arrived at unexpected creativity, immediacy and intimacy too. Likewise Access All Areas, a theatre company of people with learning disabilities and autism in Hackney, which I co-chair, moved its governance and professional theatre-making online, defying the isolation particularly felt by our artists and communities.

The #WeShallNotBeRemoved arts movement was also born, and it was powerful. Yes, we missed the essential face-to-face connection we had fought for in the arts, but together we shared our perspectives in new and accessible ways and won through again.

And alongside this, we were party to a raft of people feeling first-hand what it is like to not have the access to things, to the world outside, to the everyday things people take for granted. There was also real hope that, if people were experiencing this, that would benefit us, as the world would have greater awareness of barriers as we moved forward post-pandemic.

It suddenly became more acceptable to have flexible working hours, to rest and recoup as a natural pattern of our locked-up working lives, which emerged in response to people developing lived experiences of debilitating illness and protracted recovery, or long Covid as we know it.

All this was sadly short-lived. Eighteen months on, as lockdown and restrictions lift, things don't feel quite as hopeful.

There is a pervading fatigue, with our best warriors worn out, me included, and a real threat again to equitability, where it is no longer safe for all of us to take part and the extra resourcing for access and travel is deemed unnecessary, since we have proved we can still work without it.

And, as I sit inside, with all restrictions lifted, waiting for political motivation rather than seeing what may still be needed to ensure disabled people can still be part of the game, I feel a sense of deflation and disquiet.

We need people to remember what it felt like first-hand during those first lockdown months and to be allies with us to fight our corner as a fundamental right to ensure a representative arts future for all.

Welcome to our world
Iona Fabian

In the community of people living with ME and other disabilities, life has in many ways expanded, thanks to Covid. Already unable to leave their homes, or only occasionally, suddenly we found the world coming to us. We could attend concerts and the theatre in our own homes; our families set up regular Zoom calls, and many other activities suddenly developed online. The hope is these discoveries will mean that in the future there remains an online presence for those of us unable to attend events in person and that life will remain much more connected and interesting for everyone. Covid has been an eye-opening glimpse into how life could be.

Commentary
Patrick Vernon

The stories in this section reflect back at us a much wider issue than simply how many people were affected by (and continue to be affected by) the coronavirus. They highlight the inequalities that the headline statistics conceal: the fact that black, Asian and racialised communities, disabled people, disadvantaged people and the underclass were, as always, disproportionately affected by the virus, and yet their experience continues to be obscured and ignored. They also draw into this spotlight people who were made vulnerable because they still had to work, to make a living.

This section also speaks for asylum seekers, the homeless, people in prison, vulnerable young mothers – the truly marginalised who are mostly totally overlooked because often they have no voice, unless someone speaks for them.

And we are not in the same boat because of the structural discrimination that upholds racism, sexism and ableism in society. All these different experiences described here tell us why we need to have strong equality legislation, as inscribed in the Equalities Act of 2010, setting out in law the imperative to protect the human rights of people who belong to its nine protected categories. And it reflects the importance of intersectionality, because so many of those who come under the protection of one of those nine also fit the criteria of others. Intersectionality is really the story of Covid-19 in Britain because the existing structural issues and oppressions that many people already faced, those multiple experiences of discrimination, were then overlaid by the disproportionate effect of Covid-19, magnifying its impact.

At the end of March 2022 more than 189,000 of our loved ones had died of Covid,[2] and by 6 April 2022 more than 21 million people in the UK had tested positive with the virus.[3]

When you drill down beneath these headline figures, the data for black, Asian and minority communities in the UK are shocking. Some 21% of all healthcare staff who work for the NHS are black, Asian or minority ethnic, yet more than 63% of these workers died of Covid. When you look at nursing alone, 20% of all nursing staff are black, Asian or minority ethnic, but again, 64% of them died of Covid. The figures are even higher for doctors: 95% of black, Asian and minority ethnic doctors died, even though they represent 44% of medical staff (BMA, 2021).

Our very first story in this chapter is about Dr Gamal Osman, a GP, who died of Covid at Bristol Royal Infirmary and whose dedicated life reflects the stories of many clinicians, doctors and nurses working on the frontline, exposed to Covid by our government because they were not given the necessary protection.

And more widely, we need to remember those South-East and East Asian families and those from Turkish/Kurdish, Orthodox Jewish, African and Caribbean communities, who were not able to

---

2. https://coronavirus.data.gov.uk/details/deaths

3. https://coronavirus.data.gov.uk/details/cases

adopt the government's social isolation policies because of their housing circumstances.

What makes these data even harder to read is that the government even attempted at one point to convince the public that these deaths were somehow the fault of those who died, by suggesting there might be a genetic predisposition in these communities. This was further reinforced by the Commission on Race and Ethnic Disparities (CRED), which totally ignored the possibility that such disproportionate deaths were due to structural racial inequality, stating:

> … when examining the overall health of the UK population, it is also evident that there is more than one story to tell… life expectancy, or overall mortality, shows that ethnic minorities do better overall than the White population and actually have better outcomes for many of the 25 leading causes of death. (Commission on Race and Ethnic Disparities, 2021, p.12)

The report has been heavily criticised by NHS leaders, public health experts, race equality organisations and families who lost loved ones to Covid (Covid Families for Justice, 2021).

Michael Marmot, one of the world's leading public health experts and Director of the Institute of Healthy Equity, roundly criticised the CRED report, spelling out how it failed to recognise the cumulative effects of years of austerity on inequalities in the UK:

> . . . it was clear from the beginning of the pandemic that it would expose the underlying inequalities in society and amplify them. And then of course the pandemic makes the inequalities worse… I think of health as a measure of societal success. Pre-pandemic, life expectancy was stalling, inequalities were increasing, and life expectancy for the poorest people was falling. And during the pandemic we had the highest excess mortality. What's the link? I suggest . . . poor governance and political culture, increasing social and economic inequalities, the reduction in spending on public services. (Iacobucci, 2021)

The CRED report was used to blame and gaslight people of colour, instead of throwing light on the structural issues of racism and poverty that underlay the pandemic's inequalities. That is why the public inquiry into the Covid pandemic needs to ensure that the issue of race and other protected characteristics is fully acknowledged.

Another theme illustrated in these stories is that of community trauma. We read the story of Dame Jocelyn Barrow (p.45), who was an icon in the black community and the first black woman to be a governor of the BBC. She was a trailblazer from the Windrush generation. Her 90th birthday, which happened before lockdown at the South African High Commission, was attended by several hundred people.

Little did we know that that was the last time we would see her alive. And little did those of us who attended know that we would not see each other again for a long time because of lockdown. The account here from Dr Yansie Rolston highlights the community aspects of grief, loss and mourning. But it touches more deeply: that, when someone is obviously significant, a hero in their community, but is not white, middle-class and male, they do not get the same recognition of their contribution and how they died. That is one of the reasons I set up the Majonzi Fund[4] during lockdown, to provide small grants to families, faith groups and community organisations from black and racialised communities to acknowledge and commemorate the lives of those who died of Covid during 2020/22.

The issue around identity and belonging is raised here by Limor, a woman of colour, in the context of Covid-19, the murder of George Floyd in America and the consequent conversation in Britain about race equality, microaggressions, allyship and British colonial history. She writes (p.47) about the role of social media in this and how, to try to preserve her wellbeing because of the toxicity and negativity during this period, she disengaged from these platforms. She describes 'a psychic violence experienced by people who are affected by issues that others can't empathise with.' She powerfully speaks to the impact of racism and trauma and its magnification during Covid.

Another story is from Rahila Gupta (p.48), who talks about a couple awaiting the decision on their immigration status who might have starved without Southall Black Sisters' help, because the wife was too weak with Covid to walk to the Gurdwara, where free meals were being provided to the community. The impact of Covid-19 on women

---

4. www.majonzi-fund.com

is still to be explored, and why so many of those with long Covid are female, although there has been initial research (Suleman, 2021).

Another issue is around the impact of Covid-19 on asylum seekers. And as we know, the sympathy for asylum seekers in the UK depends heavily on their ethnicity and nationality. Refugees fleeing the Russian invasion in Ukraine are welcomed with open arms, but black and brown asylum seekers get a very different reception. When Covid struck and lockdown was instituted, no one gave a thought to the asylum seekers trapped in hostels, unable to buy food online with their prepaid cards that can only be used in person in shops. Here is Nawaf, someone else who nearly starved because he had no status as a citizen (p.49), according to the social system – and yet Britain claims to be a country that welcomes refugees and people seeking asylum.

And there are stories here showing how we did open our eyes to the lives of people we rarely see when life goes on as normal. There is the GP who worked with homeless people and went out of her clinic to meet them where they lived, because of Covid (p.50). And she noticed how one man was feeding the birds and animals because their usual source of food – waste from park users – had dried up because of Covid. 'It was the kindest thing I think I have seen in a really long time,' she writes.

Another example is the work of a girls and young women's project in Gateshead (p.56), where the workers were supporting vulnerable young girls aged just 12–19, some of them pregnant and alone. The story gives a new take on the term 'care package' – the workers were delivering boxes full of 'pamper stuff' – things that would help these isolated young women and their families feel special and taken care of. But they were also sitting on their doorsteps to talk to the young women, which was so vital, in particular to those who were pregnant and facing giving birth with no one they knew around them.

Food banks have been a key feature of the pandemic – their massive expansion, as well as that of community kitchens, and how the working poor – an invisible group for most of us, most of the time – really struggled when their income dried up. Then there were the self-employed domestic workers who, because of the pandemic, were not able to work for private clients in cleaning their homes. Clare Bateman's story graphically illustrates their vulnerability (p.61): 'My trouble is that I don't qualify for any government help because of the number of hours I work. I have an autistic son and I cannot work full time. But we need that income. We have ended up £2000 in debt.' Gordon Knott (p.53) lists vividly the ways in which the already very poor became even poorer under Covid and the disproportionate impact that has had on the young people with whom he works and their future opportunities.

In this chapter we can read several stories of people with disabilities and neurodiversity of varied kinds. It was deeply shocking when we discovered that 'do not resuscitate measures' were being used on those who were unable to give informed consent, without the agreement of carers and loved ones. During the first period of lockdown in 2020, a government report revealed that 451 per 100,000 people registered as having a learning disability died with Covid-19 between 21 March and 5 June – a death rate 4.1 times higher than the general population.[5] The pandemic was used as a reason to take away their human rights and dignity. Yet on the front line, carers and support workers did all they could to support individuals to retain a degree of dignity, personhood and quality of life, as Katie Peacock relates (p.55). And then there are those like Kenny (p.56), whose lives dwindled and were finally extinguished because of the deprivation of just being with people and out and about in the sun, which had been so key to their wellbeing.

Ironically, because the majority of people could no longer access what they were used to enjoying, lockdown turned out to be of benefit for those previously excluded – the expansion of the online world was a huge blessing for disabled people. It brought them a strange kind of equity with non-disabled people as everyone was accessing arts and cultural events and conducting their social lives online, in their own homes. The fear now for many disabled people, activists and campaigners in the disability arts world who flourished during this time is that we will go back to the old world, where the doors are slammed in their faces again and there is exclusion and discrimination. At least for a short while, Covid brought that degree of equity (pp.62–65).

The pandemic has also thrown up the whole issue of choice around taking the vaccine, which feels similar to the divide we had in the country around Brexit (p.58). Did people have the right to choose

---

5. www.gov.uk/government/publications/covid-19-deaths-of-people-with-learning-disabilities

not to take the vaccine, based on their research and rights, when not to do so threatened the effectiveness of the vaccination campaign? The experience described here is one of marginalisation and a re-evaluation of lifestyles and friendship circles, which does not fit the media narrative about anti-vaxxers.

Another powerful experience to come through strongly is that of poverty, particularly for those who were self-employed, who were another group initially overlooked by the government. Many were not entitled to the furlough scheme or business loans. People with compromised health were forced to find ways to function as best they could and, like the complementary therapist in these pages (p.60), devised their own ways of managing risk so they could continue working when there was no government guidance. Single parent families have been particularly challenged and, as Gingerbread, the charity supporting them, states, they are twice as likely to be living in poverty compared with two-parent families.[6] There have been 1,000,000 new claimants for Universal Credit since lockdown and pressure on the government to remove the five-week waiting time before the first payment. The campaign to maintain free school meals during lockdown was supported by many charities tackling poverty, as for many children it is a vital provision.

As this section illustrates, we are not in the same boat, despite what many would like to believe or pretend. There are many different boats, from ocean liners to leaky dinghies. Some boats sank or ran aground and were stranded. Some were crushed by indifferent supertankers. Some had no anchor to hold them steady and drifted onto the rocks. And some boats were already near to sinking, which meant the people in them had to work twice as hard to stay afloat.

For some people, Covid opened their eyes to the previously invisible lives of people less fortunate and protected than them, and that is good. But for many others, the pandemic simply intensified their unacknowledged struggles to survive in Britain in the 21st century. And those struggles continue today. Whether you are the hard-pressed health worker, the invisible frontline worker, the refugee facing deportation or the working family on the breadline, life looks set to get much harder and harsher for the foreseeable future.

---

6. www.gingerbread.org.uk/policy-campaigns/living-standards-and-poverty

References

BMA. (2021). *COVID-19: The risk to BAME doctors.* [Online.] BMA. www.bma.org.uk/advice-and-support/covid-19/your-health/covid-19-the-risk-to-bame-doctors

Commission on Race and Ethnic Disparities (CRED). (2021). *Commission on Race and Ethnic Disparities: The report.* CRED. https://assets.publishing.service.gov.uk/government/uploads/system/uploads/attachment_data/file/974507/20210331_-_CRED_Report_-_FINAL_-_Web_Accessible.pdf

Covid Families for Justice. (2021). *Learn lessons, save lives: What does the Covid-19 public inquiry need to include?* Covid Families for Justice. https://covidfamiliesforjustice.org/wp-content/uploads/2021/11/Learn-Lessons-Save-Lives-Final.pdf

Iacobucci, G. (2021, April 22). Covid-19: Government race review 'misused evidence', says Marmot. *BMJ, 373:* n1063. www.bmj.com/content/373/bmj.n1063

Suleman, M. (2021, April 7). *Gender divide: A post-COVID recovery must address pandemic inequalities.* [Blog.] The Health Foundation. www.health.org.uk/news-and-comment/blogs/gender-divide-a-post-covid-recovery-must-address-pandemic-inequalities

Patrick is Independent Non-Executive Director of Birmingham and Solihull ICS, where he leads on inequalities, Chair of Walsall Together Partnership, Specialist Adviser for Voice at The Centre for Ageing Better, and Chair of Citizenship Partnership for HSIB. Patrick is also a broadcaster and writes blogs and articles for the national and international media on healthcare, cultural heritage and race. He was awarded an OBE in 2012 for his work on tackling health inequalities and ethnic minority communities. In 2020 Patrick established the Majonzi Fund with Ubele, which is providing small grants to families and community organisations to organise commemoration events for individuals from black and racialised communities who have died of Covid-19. In August 2021, Patrick was appointed Honorary Professor of Cultural Heritage and Community Leadership in the Department of Community Development at Wolverhampton University.

Resources

Black, brown and minority ethnic communities

Amina: The Muslim Women's Resource Centre. An inclusive organisation that empowers and supports Muslim and BME women to create an inclusive Scotland in which they can contribute fully. *https://mwrc.org.uk*

BLAM UK. Promotes positive dialogue of social identity and culture through history, including through teaching Black history at partner schools in London. *https://blamuk.org*

Southall Black Sisters. Advice, advocacy and resource centre for women experiencing violence and abuse and other forms of inequality. https:// southallblacksisters.org.uk

Zahid Mubarak Trust. Working for systemic change in the criminal justice system to ensure racial justice and support rehabilitation and (re)integration of prisoners. *https://thezmt.org*

Books and articles

DiAngelo, R. (2019). *White fragility: Why it's so hard for white people to talk about racism*. Penguin.

Khan, A. (2019). *Razia*. Unbound.

Menakem, R. (2017). *My grandmother's hands: Racialised trauma and the pathway to mending our hearts and bodies*. Central Recovery Press.

Olusoga, D. (2016). *Black and British: A forgotten history*. Pan Books.

Roy, A. (2020, April 3). Arundhati Roy: The pandemic is a portal. *Financial Times*. www.ft.com/content/10d8f5e8-74eb-11ea-95fe-fcd274e920ca

Saad, L. (2020). *Me and white supremacy: How to recognise your privilege, combat racism and change the world*. Quercus.

Younge, G. (2021, December 16). What Covid taught us about racism – and what we need to do now. *The Guardian*. www.theguardian.com/society/2021/ dec/16/systemic-racism-covid-gary-younge

People living with learning disabilities, physical disabilities or who are neurologically diverse

The Challenging Behaviour Foundation. *www.challengingbehaviour.org.uk*

Dementia UK. *www.dementiauk.org*

Learning Disability England. Working together to build a world where people with learning disabilities have good lives with equal choices and opportunities as others. *www.learningdisabilityengland.org.uk* / *www.learningdisabilityengland. org.uk/welcome/coronavirus-hub-2*

Mencap. Advice and support for Covid-19. *www.mencap.org.uk/advice-and-support/coronavirus-covid-19*

National Autistic Society. *www.autism.org.uk*

Respond. A trauma-informed organisation supporting the lives of people with learning disabilities and autism. *www.respond.org.uk*

Books, articles, reports

Cronin, P., Hardy, S., Roberts, M., Koulla-Burke, C., Mahon, DS. & Chaplin, E. (2020). *Peter & friends talk about Covid-19 and having a learning disability and/or autism.* Foundation for People with Learning Disabilities. www. learningdisabilities.org.uk/publications/peter-friends-book-about-covid-19-and-having-learning-disability-andor-autism

Hatton, C. & Hastings, R. (2020). *Coronavirus and people with learning disabilities study: The impact of the COVID-19 pandemic on people with learning disabilities and factors associated with better outcomes.* [Online.] University of Warwick. https://warwick.ac.uk/fac/soc/cedar/covid19-learningdisability/studyinformation/

Learning Disabilities Mortality Review programme. (2020). *Deaths of people with learning disabilities from COVID-19.* University of Bristol. www.bristol. ac.uk/media-library/sites/sps/leder/Deaths%20of%20people%20with%20learning%20disabilities%20from%20COVID-19.pdf

Mencap. (2020). *My health, my life: Barriers to healthcare for people with a learning disability during the pandemic.* Mencap. www.mencap.org.uk/sites/default/files/2020-12/MyHealthMyLife_COVID%20report.pdf

Public Health England. (2020). *COVID-19: Deaths of people with learning disabilities.* Gov.uk. www.gov.uk/government/publications/covid-19-deaths-of-people-with-learning-disabilities

Peer/self-advocacy support

National Network of Parent Carer Forums. *https://nnpcf.org.uk*

Self-advocacy organisations. *https://selfadvocacygroups.co.uk*

People living in poverty or facing work related challenges

Centre for Progressive Change. Supports organisations working for progressive change. *www.centreforprogressivechange.org*

Citizen's Advice. Advice and information. *www.citizensadvice.org.uk*

Community Infosource. Supports individuals, communities, and organisations to develop skills, systems, and services. *www.infosource.org.uk*

The Equality Trust. Works to dismantle structural inequalities. *https://equalitytrust.org.uk*

Excluded UK. For individuals and organisations excluded from government Covid-19 financial support. *https://excludeduk.org*

Gingerbread. Support for single parents. *www.gingerbread.org.uk*

National Debtline. Debt advice and information. *www.nationaldebtline.org*

Poverty Alliance. Working to end poverty in Scotland. *www.povertyalliance.org*

Reuse Network. Promotes recycling and re-using. *https://reuse-network.org.uk*

Stepchange. Free online debt advice. *www.stepchange.org*

The Trussell Trust. Supports the network of food banks and campaigns to end hunger in UK. *www.trusselltrust.org*

Books

Bambra, C., Lynch, J. & Smith, K.E. (2021). *The unequal pandemic: Covid-19 and health inequalities*. Policy Press.

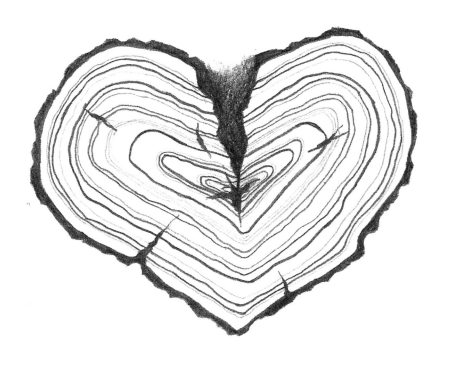

3.

Torn apart

Gone

Saying goodbye at the ambulance door, they drove him away. We couldn't visit. He died.

My neighbour died this evening

Thérèse Maitland

My neighbour died this evening. Late afternoon, lead grey skies and colder than the previous days. She must have thought, 'Better go now while the sun is not shining.'

I know she died because I saw a charcoal-grey van patiently waiting in front of their detached, single-garage house. It was slightly tilted on the curb, discreetly parked to allow neighbours to pass by and carry on with their daily activities. And when I passed, coming back from town, I saw the sober lettering in another shade of grey: Private Ambulance.

And then, as I was unloading my shopping from the car, the undertakers appeared, carrying a stretcher with a body bag, which showed just ever so slightly under the covering blanket. A sturdy, rusty, rubbery, zipped-up bag. I recognised it because I had seen one a few weeks earlier, when my husband died. They slipped the stretcher smoothly, gently, into the back of the van and closed the doors.

And six members of the family, in full compliance with the latest anti-Covid 'rule of six', stood under the porch in front of their half-open front door, all dutifully masked, and they waved as the private ambulance gently moved off. They waved goodbye to their wife, mum and sister.

Then, like a perfectly choreographed group of starlings, the group turned their back in unison to re-enter the house. That is when I heard my neighbour say something along the lines of 'Go and see her.'

And his lovely blond daughter, who also lives a few doors down, came towards me and opened her arms so wide, I could not avoid the strong and warm embrace, although my mind was in conflict because she was wearing a mask and I wasn't.

And then we cried together on my driveway. We kept repeating, 'So hard, so hard!' She told me that she waved my John goodbye when the hearse took him away on the day of his funeral. 'Goodbye, Trumpet John,' she said. He was a trumpeter, my John, and since he left, the air no longer carries Fantini's sonatas and capricci to our neighbours' windows at supper time.

Sisters forever

Jane

Gof caught Covid very early on in its trail of devastation across Great Britain. Gof was helping a friend who was bed-bound with multiple sclerosis and lived near us in Faringdon. Philip went into hospital on a Thursday and came out on Tuesday. By this time, Gof had been told by his GP on the phone, 'Oh yes, you have probably got Covid, so you need to isolate.' No other advice. He called an ambulance on the Wednesday, but the crew told him that, as he could talk in full sentences, he was okay. The next day, I called another ambulance as he was really having trouble getting his breath, and they took him to hospital. We thought he would be gone a couple of days, so he chose to go to the local hospital in Swindon. Within three hours of arrival, he was on a ventilator. Thank goodness they had a spare one, we thought. For 14 days, they rang twice a day with news, which we clung to with hope. Gof was taken off the ventilator on the Wednesday and on the Friday we were so 'lucky' to be able to go in and say goodbye to him!!! He was unaware we were there, and I had PTSD from the sound of his desperate fight for each breath. Our world changed forever. Our son Matthew and I were alone. No funeral, no contact with the outside world; we had to isolate again because we had been in the Covid ward.

Later on in that year, I joined the facilitators and seven other people on a 10-session online course for people bereaved by Covid. I was very quiet, reserved and heartbroken. It is difficult to remember those first meetings when we didn't know each other. During the meetings, it was as if John and Lynne, the facilitators, held us in their arms as we began to unwind to share the horrendous times we had all experienced. They understood, they listened, they let us tell all of the horrid, horrid things that had happened. Gently, we became an unbreakable unit that we now call Sisters Forever, and we meet via Zoom at least once a week.

Double lockdown

Basia Schofield

I lost my husband to a sudden and tragic death by suicide a couple of weeks before we entered the first Covid lockdown. Very quickly, with the unfolding crisis, I was cut off from the rest of the world – from family, friends, the local community. I wanted to organise a funeral for everyone able to come from different corners of the world (including my family, who live abroad) to grieve together. In the end, we were allowed to have only five mourners – just the closest family members – and five more for the very last moment of the burial. It was heart-breaking. I promised myself, his friends and mostly him to organise a memorial, which also had to be postponed a few times due to another lockdown or Covid-related restrictions. In a sense, it brought a closure, but it couldn't bring the whole community to mourn together, like funerals do.

As for my grief, a grief in times of a pandemic and the lockdowns, it's been a strange journey. Even more painful and lonely, due to an imposed isolation when I needed people around me the most. The cards showing sympathy were pouring through the letter box, but couldn't replace real hugs, human warmth, the reflection of my pain in someone else's eyes. But people were there for me, out there; they found ways to support me. A local friend would ask me to go for a walk every day. Another brought food every evening until the funeral, delivered to my door. Another proposed a video call every morning at 10am, when I couldn't really see a point in getting up... These wonderful, kind people really have looked after me and kept me going.

However, as my whole world turned upside down, it strangely aligned with the outside world. Both worlds – my own and the one outside of me – were abnormal. I was in a double lockdown. It turned out to be a gift. It allowed me to grieve well, as everything stopped. I could give myself a lot of space and quiet to remember, to reflect, to cry, not be sucked into the fast, busy world full of life at a time when I felt there was no life for me. I wanted to stay in this quiet place and the world around me to stay too. But life goes on, and so do I.

No touching

Deborah Lewis

Not being allowed to touch the coffin – we could only place our beautiful little posies on it and absolutely not touch the basket.

Prison sentence

Andy

Andy's wife, Lorraine, began her battle with cancer when she was 41. She had two bouts of breast cancer, and a mastectomy, but the cancer metastasised in 2019 when she was 60. It spread to her lung and then other organs. From March 2020, the lockdown meant that Lorraine had to stay at home because of the risk of getting Covid in hospital. Andy had to take over as her full-time carer.

Lorraine was suffering horrendous pain most of the time. When she wasn't in pain, she was asleep or knocked out by the strong drugs. The district nurses came every one or two days to drain her lung, which always caused yet more pain. It was a nightmare for Andy; he had no time to himself and no quality time, apart from taking the dog for a walk when Lorraine slept. For more than six months, it felt like he was living a prison sentence, he said. The one positive was that he was furloughed from work, which enabled him to do the caring. However, he was then made redundant a few weeks before Lorraine died. She was admitted to hospital at the end, as she had an infection. Andy, their daughter and Lorraine's brother were with her.

The aftermath for Andy was dreadful as he had absolutely no support from the hospital or the GP. He was broken. He considered and planned suicide because he still had all the medication. But Lorraine had said, 'Don't you do anything stupid when I'm gone.' He couldn't leave his daughter alone and he worried about what would happen to his dog.

20th May 2020

Thérèse Maitland

I feel I have to explain to our Prime Minister[1] the meaning of 'lockdown' and what happened to us and so many others who followed his laws, guided by our own moral compass and sense of social responsibility.

I don't like being angry, but I find that I am. Not against the rules but against the rule-breakers.

My beloved husband died at home, of cancer, which spread rapidly after he was diagnosed with Covid on 21st March and his immunotherapy treatments were stopped.

While Downing Street staff were taking empty suitcases to off licences to be refilled with bottles of booze, and partying into the early hours of the morning, my daughter-in-law, a nurse, was making frantic phone calls to get authorisation for additional morphine. We had run out, the day before his death.

From February to 22nd June, no doctor visited our home. We had one disheartening visit from a palliative care person, who gave no emotional support, focusing instead on explaining to me how to administer Ora-morph and keep track of every dose in a little book. I still have the book, which is the saddest document I have ever owned. My name was on a waiting list for a Macmillan night nurse, but it never made it to the top.

The district nurses were magnificent – heroic! But their availability was limited. So, while parties were being held in Downing Street to shore up the courage of politicians and government workers, I, a 73-year-old woman, who had recently undergone a mastectomy for breast cancer, was queuing, fully masked, outside a dispensary window to collect morphine. Friends could not come to our home to help or put the kettle on, although many left home-cooked food at the door and lovely notes of comfort. One of my husband's best friends 'broke the rule' for just a few hours. He needed to say goodbye. And you know what? We felt so guilty about that infraction!

On my own, I changed my husband's stoma, drained his lung into sterile bottles that were dropped off and picked up at the door,

---

1. Boris Johnson was Prime Minister at the time of writing. He subsequently resigned, in part because of his attendance at parties for staff at Downing Street that were deemed to have broken lockdown rules.

changed his bed and cleaned him. On the last day of May, I asked one of our sons to come into the house to help. From then on, he stayed with us in isolation until the end.

And many were much less privileged than I – their loved ones were taken away from them to die on their own.

This is the meaning of lockdown, Mr. Johnson! While you are redefining the meaning of the words 'party' and 'work meeting', some of us are reliving the utter loneliness and abandonment of the last days of our loved ones.

When Peter Pan died
Emma

As we approach my second Father's Day without my dad, I feel kind of cheated now – cheated for so many reasons, but mainly because, at the core of this all, he did not need to die – he was taken away from us unnecessarily.

My dad will always be 77 – he was a young 77 and we always called him Peter Pan – his name was Peter and he never grew up. In fact, that was part of the reason I was not talking to him when he died. I am the eldest of three, and was always a daddy's girl, but I had had to make a decision two-and-a-half years previously to walk away from his dramas, for the sake of my own health, and that in itself has been so very hard for me to deal with, along with everything we already know about the complex grief process that is going on at the moment.

He left us on 2nd April 2020 – 24 hours after my son found him hallucinating and barely conscious. What went on in those 24 hours I hope nobody I know ever has to go through – it might sound strange, but I feel lucky in a way that I did not have to deal with days of waiting, days of not knowing what was going on – I had just 24 hours. I was also fortunate that the hospital called me every hour, not with an update on how his progress was, because they had already told me that he would not make it through the night, but to tell me he was still alive. They also said that one family member could go to the hospital and Oli, my son, who had already been with him so therefore had to isolate, made the brave decision to do so – he sat with him for an hour while we all said our goodbyes over the phone.

My dad died at 6pm on 2nd April without any of us being with him. He was Jewish, and in our religion we are meant to bury people within

24 hours where possible, so I did what I knew best – I threw myself into 'sorting things out' and was able to arrange the death certificate and burial for the Sunday, not quite 24 hours but the cemetery and the local council were so overwhelmed at that time, it was the best we could do. I should not have gone because of my high risk, but there was no way I was going to have my dad buried without me.

What ensued over the next few months I cannot put into words – every emotion going; every part of me wanted answers; every part of me felt guilt, anger, hate; but as I have had mental health problems in the past, I knew I had to accept these feelings and use all my coping mechanisms to keep me going, when in truth there were times when I felt like I actually couldn't.

The Covid ward
Carole

My experience of losing my mum will be forever etched in my mind. She went into hospital with a urinary tract infection and was knowingly put on a ward where Covid was rife 'because there's nowhere else to put her'. She tested positive the third time. Several horrendous days followed of her getting worse and me trying to talk to her on the phone. Listening to her saying, 'I'm scared, Caj, but I love you.' Never hearing those words again. Then the doctor ringing me to say we need to put a Do Not Resuscitate in place, to which I said no because mum had made it clear that she wanted to be revived. The doctor arguing with me about it and then deciding to put her in end-of-life care without any input from me. So my thoughts and feelings were irrelevant. I accused him of euthanasia, to which he told me that there was no choice. 'Oh, she'll probably last a few days.' She went the next morning, with no warning. I will always feel that the decision to place her on a Covid ward when she didn't have it ultimately ended her life prematurely, and I can never forgive that. I'll miss you forever, beautiful Mum. xx

Orphaned by Covid
Marie Francoise Rosat

My younger brother, Jean Luc Rosat, was 67 years old and lived in Rio de Janeiro. He had been a well-known athlete in the 70s, playing volleyball in the national team and representing Brazil twice in the

Olympics. He was a father and grandfather, and was still working as the manager of a well-known restaurant.

He often played volleyball at the beach on Sundays, and tennis during the week. I had the belief that someone who does lots of sport outdoors must have a good immune system. At the beginning of March 2020, he started to feel ill, coughing a lot, and eventually got fever, so he thought he had flu. After some days, he decided to get a PCR test and discovered that he had Covid. His family doctor thought it could be risky for him to go to the hospital, as in Rio all the hospitals were at breaking point with so many seriously ill patients. Then he started to have difficulty in breathing and he needed oxygen. He was lucky enough to find a private clinic where he got very good care. Despite this, he went into intensive care two days later, had to be intubated and was put in an artificial coma. Two weeks later, after getting better and then worse, he had cerebral bleeding and died. All this time no one in the family could visit him. His two sons met the doctors in the hospital car park for updates on their father. Because I do not live in Brazil, I could only communicate via WhatsApp. None of us could say goodbye to him. We were all separated, and he died alone. It was horrible.

Yet on the television they observed a minute's silence before starting their volleyball matches. It was very moving to see all these young men and women honouring my own brother in front of his picture on a huge screen in the stadium. I watched all that from afar, with my broken heart and a mixture of pride and sadness.

My parents died before all this. All three all gone, and I am the elder and survivor. I feel like an orphan right now. It aches every day.

I will always be grateful for having had them in my life until I was almost 70 years old. And life goes on. I will mourn at my own pace, letting my heart mend the broken pieces.

The wall of grief and love

Fran Hall

I find myself here at the wall because the man I loved and lived with for more than 11 years, and then married, contracted Covid and was dead within three weeks of that happy day in September 2020.

Our wall stretches for more than 500 metres along the Albert Embankment. Formerly a cream stone wall bounding the perimeter of St. Thomas' Hospital, from a distance it now looks blood red. Close up, this red wall reveals itself to be comprised of hundreds of thousands of individual hearts, each painted by hand, each one representing one person who died with Covid-19 on their death certificate. It takes almost 10 minutes to walk the length of it, much longer if you pause to read some of the heart-breaking dedications written in the hearts.

The wall is maintained by a small group of dedicated volunteers. We meet each week to remove graffiti, refresh existing hearts and add inscriptions on behalf of bereaved families from around the UK.

All of us are women, all personally bereaved by Covid. We volunteers have become close friends in our shared grief and our shared determination that those who died in such horrendous circumstances – often alone, without family around them, struggling for breath and terrified – will not be forgotten, and that the scale of the loss suffered by this country – one of the worst in the world – will be understood.

'I will never stop coming here,' said one of our group, who travels down from the West Midlands every Friday. 'As long as I am physically capable, I'll be at the wall every week. This is what has helped me survive. Without the wall, I don't know how I would have got through this. It is horrific, what has happened to us. Utterly horrific.'

So far, there has been no official recognition of this catastrophic death toll, no national mourning or remembrance. Our pain feels invisible as the government pushes a narrative of 'moving on'. But there is this unofficial one, created by bereaved families in early April 2021, in an audacious act of determination that those lost to the pandemic will not be wiped from history. The National Covid Memorial Wall stands in silent rebuke to those in power, directly across the Thames from the Palace of Westminster, reminding us all of the more than 200,000 deaths and the failures of those who were supposed to keep us safe.

Haunted

Tony

I lost my wife Ann on the 7th April 2020. We had been soulmates for 47 years. Ann left home at 16, held down a full-time day job, worked in bars while under age, telling the owners she was 18. She was a stunner. All my mates kept asking, 'How did you pull her?' She had a tough upbringing. None of her family came to our wedding. We had a bond so strong because of what she'd been through; we were inseparable.

Not only am I struggling with the loss, it's the way that it happened that I am really having difficulty in understanding and accepting. Ann and I had all the classic symptoms of Covid, and for 10 days we just accepted that we had to self-isolate at home. On the 11th day Ann was really struggling, but prior to that, she never once said she thought she needed any medical help. I called an ambulance on the morning of the 11th day and even the paramedics didn't seem overly concerned and thought she might need antibiotics but she would be better being checked over at our local hospital. We assumed she would be there for a few hours and then I would receive a call to collect her. I never thought for one moment that it would be the last time I would ever see her. I never even had the chance to give her a kiss or a hug, and she just said, 'I'll ring you later' and got into the ambulance.

Sadly, she passed away. The fact she was not allowed to see me or our children haunts me. My daughter cries, saying she never had a chance to speak to or say 'bye to her mum. Before Ann passed away, she managed to message me saying she thought that she wasn't going to make it and regretting that she hadn't written farewell letters to me and our children and that she wished we could be there with her. That haunts me as well; it's horrendous. I can't get it out of my mind of how lonely and frightened Ann must have been. I will never forget any of that and it's with me every single day.

We can always see her later in the year

Anna

My mother was in a care home when Covid-19 hit. We were due to go see her just as lockdown began but cancelled due to concerns for her safety. 'We can always see her later in the year,' we thought. We felt reassured the care home was keeping her as protected as possible.

Unfortunately, that 'later' never came. As the wave hit in December 2020, most of the residents caught the virus, including my mother. The care home housed the frailest residents. We always knew the outcome would be devastating when the virus hit. It was like waiting for a ticking bomb to go off.

When we had the call that Mum had caught Covid-19, it became a waiting game. We tried to keep hopeful that she would be one of the lucky ones that the virus wouldn't affect too much (we knew it was a long shot, but you grasp at whatever you can), but after a few days she was deteriorating, and they sent her to hospital.

I can't really explain how isolating it is having a loved one in hospital during the pandemic, both for the patient and for those waiting. My mother was alone and, due to her dementia, she had no idea what was going on. It felt like an insurmountable chasm between where she lay and where we were at home. We'd hear snippets of what was happening to her in a call each day from the hospital, but you feel detached from the whole situation and completely helpless.

I'm ever-thankful to one of the kind nurses who took the time to sit with her and then talk me through her time with Mum – how Mum was curled up comfortably in her blankets, how the nurse had left the window open a crack to let some fresh air in for her. It made me feel I was there and could see her.

Mum only lasted a few days; she was too frail for the options they had on ICU. I like to tell myself her passing was peaceful, and in a way it was. She went to sleep for a couple of days and never woke up. But I think that's making it sound easy.

I really struggled to process Mum's death initially. Not being able to be with her, hold her hand, not being able to see her body – I can almost convince myself that she is still with us. Even registering her death and arranging her funeral remotely just seemed unreal.

I found the funeral the hardest, with only five of us attending. Afterwards, it was a bit of an abyss. I joined a Facebook group, and it was good to share stories with others who had been in the same situation. I then joined a weekly group session over Zoom, where a few of us could share our experiences and support each other. I found this a massive comfort. Instead of not knowing what to do with myself, I had a safe space each week that let me share my thoughts and feelings. It allowed me to work through my grief at a time when I would have really struggled with finding an outlet.

Making meaning
Lindsay Jackson

My mum was suffering from dementia. She was diagnosed in 2017 and I took early retirement to look after her. She had Lewy body dementia, and she had a lot of hallucinations. At the start she was fine with them; she knew they were hallucinations and she was seeing people she loved – my dad, her brothers, her own mum and dad. But then they got frightening. She thought people were trying to kill her, and her reaction was to try to get away, and she was running out of the house at all hours of the day and night and putting herself in danger. So I found a nice residential home, and she moved in there in December 2019 and settled in quite quickly. She didn't know where she was, but I spent three or fours hours a day with her. She was an actor and theatre director, and she loved music. So we would spend the time just singing.

Then Covid came and lockdown on 23 March 2020, and I couldn't see her after, except on Skype, which worked okay as I'd been abroad a lot and we'd Skyped, so she knew it was me. But then I got a call saying they'd got Covid in the home and I knew it was a matter of when, not if Mum got it. They called me on Friday 10 April to say she'd got a cough and they'd called 111 and been advised to treat it as Covid. I saw Mum on Skype and I could see her temperature was very high – her face was flushed and she was delirious. With dementia, you only need a smidgeon of infection and everything goes chaotic. She was very distressed, so they sedated her.

She never saw a doctor; the district nurses were taking in the drugs and after two days they suggested a syringe driver. It was explained to me that this was it; this would be the end; she'd be sedated to the end of her life. I'd already said I didn't want her admitted to hospital.

She died a week after she contracted Covid. The home had told me I could go and see her just for five minutes to say goodbye before she died; and I didn't feel that was right, because it wasn't what the government regulations were saying. However, on 16th April the government said that people could go into residential homes to say goodbye – so I did go and see her.

I donned all my own PPE – cagoule, waterproof trousers, goggles, dust mask – I didn't want to use the PPE at the care home. I think she knew I was in the room but she was very heavily sedated – there was a little movement of her mouth that made me think she knew it was me. I just stood at a distance and spoke to her and said goodbye and came away. I didn't touch her; I didn't know if I could do that. And she died the following evening. I was told she wasn't on her own when she died, which was some comfort.

There were just seven of us at her funeral and it was a very short service because they were limiting the time so they could clean everything and get more people through, to be brutally honest. And after, we couldn't hug or anything. We just all got back in our cars and drove off to our respective homes. It was a nice day, so my husband and I sat in the garden and talked about Mum, but it made me realise how important that gathering after a funeral is. It leaves you in the air if you don't have it – you don't have the chance to reminisce or put the death into place so you can move on. It felt like she was just taken from us and we couldn't accompany her on her journey.

Then, when I heard about the antics at Downing Street, and how the civil servants and Boris Johnson were breaking the lockdown rules, it made me feel at some level that I let her down: that if I hadn't followed these stupid rules that even the government didn't follow, she wouldn't have left this life on her own. I felt an idiot. But also, it triggered something. It's not a nice experience to sit by the bed of someone who is dying – I did it with my dad. I have a sneaking feeling that, because the government said I couldn't be with her, it took the responsibility from me, and maybe I didn't want to. I would have, but I have a sneaking feeling that part of me was relieved that I didn't have to be there and that makes me feel guilty.

What's happened hasn't stopped me living my life, but I think about her every day – probably every hour: not always sadly, but when I have to think about what happened to her, I'm right back there and it's very raw. I joined the campaign Covid-19 Bereaved Families for Justice because I feel that, if the inquiry we've been pressing for leads to positive change and we learn from this pandemic and are better prepared for the next one that is sure to come, I will have done something to give her death some meaning.

We were finally able to have a church ceremony to bury her ashes in August 2021. After, we had a huge celebration of her life at a posh hotel, with afternoon tea and a brass band and fellow actors singing and performing. It was a proper send off – 100 people came. She would have loved it.

Why I can't grieve

Jo Goodman, Co-Founder of Covid-19 Bereaved Families for Justice

Covid just swoops in and robs you of your life and the deaths keep coming and the numbers seem weirdly normalised as we read them each day. It's very hard because I spend the majority of the time dealing with the fact my dad died of Covid, not that he died. I will not be able to properly grieve until there has been a statutory public inquiry with a rapid review phase and we know when and why decisions were taken and what we can learn to prevent events like this happening again.

Giving birth in a pandemic
Sophie McManus

Our first child was born in the first lockdown. All the birthing books and classes talk about birth as a primal instinctive process, saying the best way you can aid its progression is to make sure you are in a familiar surroundings with someone you trust. You're also told this is all vital to reduce the risk of medical intervention. So we had hoped for a home birth. People give accounts, laughing about how they went from seven centimetres dilated to zero in two minutes when faced with a gruff doctor's examination. Imagine if you can the terror, after learning the above, of being told you had to deliver in a building you'd never seen, without anyone you knew present.

Secure in the knowledge that all was well and that I didn't need a scan, as my midwives had told me, I ended up at 42 weeks on my own in hospital listening to my baby's heart rate drop before being rushed into an emergency C-section. I am lucky that my husband arrived in the nick of time to come in with me to the theatre, lucky they let him in at all, as not all hospitals did. We had two hours together. I don't remember much of it because I was woozy from the surgery. After that, no one was there with me and my son to celebrate, to change his first poo, to care for us or make me laugh. I needed help. I managed to get discharged at 9pm the day after by crying and threatening to walk out without my papers. Then those survival hormones faded and I was left with daunting flashbacks.

Fast forward, and I'm working from home, managing my own business, and my husband is going back to the office next week after almost two years of being there every day with me and our baby – driving me to appointments, holding my hand, sharing the load. The best possible start for our son, and for my new business. It can't take away the trauma of birthing my first child in a pandemic, but my goodness, don't I just know how much it has helped me to get through.

Struggling[2]

Really struggling.

Not being able to see him is very frustrating. Phoning him up occasionally

to try and have a conversation with him because you can guess how he really is

a bit better than them just saying he's fine.

You know, actually to hear his voice?

Connection[2]

Connection has changed over time. The home mum is in is fantastic in regard to care, hygiene, nutrition and so on, but not when it comes to remote conversations and tech. Mum hasn't been able to talk just on the phone, not since she moved into the home. What we ended up doing for the most of last year was to rely on individual carers who happened to have Apple phones, and for them to Facetime me so I could actually have a conversation with my mother.

The very first time that I did a Facetime call with her, she clearly did connect with me; she still recognised my voice then. As well as fairly advanced dementia, my mum also has macular degeneration, but certainly a year ago she recognised my voice at least and really knew that it was me who was calling.

The end of the call consisted of her taking the phone from the carer and literally smacking her lips against it, so I saw my mum's face appearing right up close to the camera and it was – well, it made me cry, that kiss… it was just wonderful. It was really, really precious.

You can't come in, Gran

Barbara Welford

Our living situation is unusual. We live in a small hamlet, based around a farm. We have six houses within a few hundred metres of each other, containing 16 family members spanning four generations. When the lockdown measures were announced in March 2020, we

---

2. These two contributions are from *A Little Bit of Magic: Care home conversations in Covid times*, curated and edited by Pippa Marriott for the All is Mended project.

regrouped ourselves into 'bubbles' in order to provide the necessary childcare support. This meant that my elderly parents-in-law were left with only indirect support because bubbles could consist of only two households. We bubbled instead with our son and his family, who needed the childcare support, the local nursery having shut and my son and his wife being essential workers.

My mother-in-law continued to walk up and down the road, calling in at the family homes, as she had always done. She found herself greeted with 'You can't come in, Gran'. Every time this was said to her, it appeared to be a surprise. She voiced the opinion that surely the rules didn't really apply to us in our hamlet and that she didn't mind if she got Covid.

It seems to me that this enforced separation from close family support began a deterioration in her mental health. She became anxious and demanding and self-absorbed. On our part, it was hard to maintain sympathy and patience with her in the face of her constant complaints about the hardships she was facing when the very real isolation and difficulties endured by many others was on the news every day.

Commentary

Lynne Gabriel and John Wilson

The stories in this section are a cross-section of what has become a familiar narrative to those who work in this arena – the health and care workers, the funeral directors, religious leaders, social workers and counsellors. We could hardly have imagined such accounts before Covid struck. People who fell ill with breathing difficulties were taken away by ambulance with a 'See you later' wave, rapidly deteriorated and died soon after. A few 'lucky' families were able to say goodbye, but dressed in gowns, masks and gloves. Such was the fear and level of precaution that bodies were quickly sealed in coffins to prevent infection, and the bereaved were denied time to sit in the chapel of rest with their loved ones. Funerals were truncated, music was not allowed, the coffin was placed out of reach for fear of mourner cross-infection. Overstretched NHS staff were not always able to communicate adequately with relatives anxious for updates. Belongings, even jewellery, occasionally got lost. Yet there were also numerous accounts of health workers going the extra mile, holding video phones to their dying patient so that those who loved them could say goodbye. There were stories of compassionate funeral directors bending the rules, of socially distanced communities lining funeral routes. We know that these human touches made a difference.

These stories speak for themselves. Some of them come from the members of a closed social media group we opened soon after the Covid-19 pandemic begun, which we'll describe further below.

Thérèse's observation of the death of a neighbour, written with the empathy of somebody who had gone through the death of her own husband a few weeks earlier, also discreetly carried away in a 'rusty, rubbery' body bag, is truly moving (p.77). And, as we tend to do here in the UK, the family, in their darkest moments of desperation, still observed the Covid rules of masks and social distancing as they watched the ambulance begin its sad journey to the mortuary.

Jane's story (p.78) is similar to those we heard many times. Unlike many in Jane's situation, she and her son were able to be at her husband's bedside at the end of his life, and we can hope that he had an idea that they were there.

Basia's story (p.79) demonstrates starkly that the lockdown had equally devastating effects on those experiencing a bereavement that was not Covid-related during the pandemic. Death by suicide is one of the worst ways to lose a loved one, and the funeral Basia had hoped for could have gone some way to mitigating her family's grief. A funeral is a time-honoured ritual where the family comes together to honour and to eulogise. The emotional and physical contact helps in ways that are difficult to understand unless you have been there. To have that taken away – to be permitted only a small, restricted funeral – was, as Basia says, 'heart-breaking'. It is a story we have heard many times from our group members. Yet Basia was able to find solace in the quiet of lockdown – space to grieve deeply and intensely, free from a normally busy world. Perhaps we have something to learn from those cultures who grant widows time and space to grieve.

Deborah's brief and poignant comment (p.80) about not even being allowed to touch the coffin encapsulates what we have heard so often – a fear of the virus and its unknown characteristics, which for many months made it necessary to have such harsh rules. We have been very aware of the emotional harm caused by these, albeit understandable, restrictions.

Andy's experience of supporting his dying wife through the pandemic, denied palliative care because of the risks of Covid, is similarly heart-breaking (p.80). Although furlough had a positive side to it, because it gave him time off work to care for Lorraine, the ensuing redundancy would have been a stress that added to his grief and anxiety. It seems so sad that Andy was left contemplating suicide and feeling there was nobody to reach out to. In the end, his life was saved by his love and promise to Lorraine.

Thérèse echoes the justifiable anger of so many who struggled to manage their partner's illness within the rules, while those who made the rules partied (p.81). We hope, for Thérèse's sake, and for the sake of all the others who felt unsupported in delivering end-of-life care to their partner, that genuine lessons will be learned.

Emma (p.82) had enough integrity and awareness of her self-care needs to distance herself from her Peter-Pan dad's behaviour, yet she was there for him at the end as much as she could be. We know that, through creating this continuing bond, she has a new and loving relationship that will endure forever.

How do you rebuild your life knowing that your mother was put onto a ward with Covid patients when she was admitted to hospital for another reason? How do you recover from believing that, to all intents and purposes, your mother was euthanised? Somehow, with the support of friends, family and professionals, Carole (p.83) is slowly rebuilding her life.

Covid grief has been universal, and the effects have stretched across nations, as families have been separated through living in different parts of the world. How would we have coped without modern technology to communicate with families? It must have been at least some comfort for Jean Luc Rosat's sister to see his life celebrated on Brazilian television (p.83). We know that recognition of a life by wider public can be a comfort to the bereaved.

Tony's story is a familiar one (p.85). So many people during the pandemic waved their loved one off in the ambulance, never to see them again, not even in the chapel of rest. Tony knows he will never get over his loss because we grieve our loved ones for the rest of our life. We learn to live with it. All Tony has are his memories of a loving soulmate.

Some of the most tragic stories from the pandemic are the experiences of staff and residents in care homes. With inadequate personal protection equipment, so many care homes changed overnight from a safe and loving space to a place with a high risk of death. So many residents with dementia died with no understanding of what was happening, feeling abandoned by their family. How do you make meaning of that? We don't know if you can. Perhaps you have to rely on memories of better times and try to find some way to forgive yourself and others. Anna's mother (p.86) had a kind nurse who talked Anna through her mother's last hours. We know how important it is to have an account of our loved one's death, and to be able to retell this story as part of making sense of the death. Anna was also helped by being part of one of our support groups, where she could tell her story and share her emotions with others bereaved by Covid. Government restrictions eased just in time for Lindsay (p.87) to visit her dying mother, but she can only guess whether her mother knew she had come; her mother was too heavily sedated to acknowledge her presence.

And rules were also bent. When Sophie and her husband planned their baby (p.90), they could not have imagined the frightening circumstances of bringing life into a pandemic world. Yet, despite the isolation Sophie experienced, hospital staff were compassionate enough to allow her husband to be present at the birth. There was a upside in that the pandemic lockdown and home working allowed the family more time together in their baby son's first two years than would have been possible in more normal circumstances.

Online support

The Facebook support group we formed at the start of the pandemic at York St John University's counselling and mental health centre had nearly 700 members by August 2022, and it continues to provide support, alongside an online bereavement support group. The group includes counsellors and therapists and people from different cultures across the four home countries of the UK, as well from the USA. We actively sought to encourage counsellors and psychotherapists into the group, for their empathy and willingness to listen to others. Many of those who joined had been bereaved by Covid themselves, and so brought a special understanding. Members were of all ages, genders, sexual identities, religions, cultural heritages and ethnic backgrounds. Justified and legitimate exclusions aside, inclusivity was a central feature. We made the decision that members should be able to express the whole range of emotions, including anger, including towards politicians – we believed this was a valid expression of emotions.

Inclusivity has been our watchword, for all the reasons spelled out in this new member's first post:

> I'm not sure if I will be accepted in this group as I'm not sure my story is the same as everyone else's as my mum passed away from a rare form of cancer and not cov19, but during the lockdown 2020. I feel very isolated and still am in shock but first wanted to ask if I will be welcome.

She was, of course, warmly welcomed to the group.

Others joined the group because the intensity of their grief had not been recognised by friends and family, or even by members of other such groups.

> I have found in some groups, people try to say that one person's grief isn't as 'important' or 'bad' as someone else's, people comparing grief and minimising people's experiences.

And this is, of course, the power and healing potential of such a group, and more so during the pandemic when restrictions denied us all that experience of sharing with others that is so important to making meaning of a death (Neimeyer & Lee, 2022). Disenfranchisements of our right and freedom to grieve were universal during the pandemic (Albuquerque et al., 2021). The impact of pandemic loss was common to all humankind, but it was also unique to individual grievers. The pandemic heightened grief trauma in ways that we have never encountered. The traumatic separation experiences due to lockdown and infection control measures wrought a terrible toll on the bereaved. Choices about who families could invite into their 'bubble' meant some elders were excluded and became lonely and isolated, as poignantly highlighted by Barbara (p.91) in the closing story here.

Members tell us that the most important benefit of groups such as ours is the space they offer for the sharing of their stories and the recognition that you are not alone; that others are in the same or similar situation, and that how you feel is valid and worthy of sympathy and comfort. Research has repeatedly shown the value of bereaved families being able to come together to provide exactly this support and comfort, as well as memorialise the dead (Walter, 2007; McManus et al., 2018). The lockdown denied people that opportunity. Families were separated, funerals were restricted in numbers and the comfort of human touch forbidden. People were not allowed to follow important cultural rituals and practices. Members of our group, while recognising the need for restrictions, were able to share their guilt, disappointment and anger.

We are thankful for the generosity of those who told their stories here. What happened must not be forgotten, and lessons must be learnt.

References

Albuquerque, S., Teixeira, A.M. & Rocha, J.C. (2021). COVID-19 and disenfranchised grief. *Frontiers in Psychiatry, 12*. doi: 10.3389/fpsyt.2021.638874

McManus, R., Walter, T. & Claridge, L. (2018). Restoration and loss after disaster: Applying the dual-process model of coping in bereavement. *Death Studies, 42*(7), 405–414.

Neimeyer, R. & Lee, S.A. (2022). Circumstances of the death and associated risk factors for severity and impairment of COVID-19 grief. *Death Studies, 46*(1), 34–42.

Walter, T. (2007). Modern grief, postmodern grief. *International Review of Sociology – Revue Internationale de Sociologie, 17*(1), 123–134.

Lynne Gabriel is a professor of counselling and mental health and the founder and director of the York St John Communities Centre. Lynne is an active psychotherapist, teacher, researcher and supervisor. She has worked with bereaved people throughout her career in mental health and through the Centre, and facilitates bereavement support groups in collaboration with Dr John Wilson. Lynne chairs the Centre's annual International Online Bereavement Conference and presents at conferences on bereavement and other aspects of the human condition.

Dr John Wilson lives near York with wife Sandra and four cats. Now a Visiting Fellow at York St John University, he previously worked for 17 years as bereavement counsellor at St Catherine's Hospice, Scarborough. He was awarded a PhD for bereavement counselling research in 2017, since when he has directed the Bereavement Service at York St John University Communities Centre. John is the author of two books: *Supporting People through Loss and Grief: An introduction for counsellors and other caring practitioners* (2013), and *The Plain Guide to Grief* (2020). John teaches bereavement counselling theory and practice and regularly presents co-authored research with Lynne Gabriel, in articles and at international conferences. He is currently in the early stages of a third book.

Resources

See Chapter 4 'Our Future' for resources for and about bereaved young people.

Books

Borgstrom, E. & Mallon, S. (2021). *Narratives of COVID: Loss, dying, death and grief during COVID-19*. Open University Press.

Graves, D. (2009). *Talking with bereaved people*. Jessica Kingsley.

Lewis, C.S. (1961/2015). *A grief observed* (Reader's ed.). Faber & Faber.

Macdonald, H. (2014). *H is for hawk*. Jonathan Cape.

McLoighlin, J. (Ed.). (1994). *On the death of a parent*. Virago.

Porter, M. (2015). *Grief is the thing with feathers*. Faber & Faber.

Rentzenbrink, C. (2017). *Manual for heartache*. Picador.

Riley, D. (2019). *Time lived without its flow*. Picador.

Rosenfeld, J. (2020). *The state of disbelief*. Short Books.

Rothschild, L. (Ed.). (2020). *Outside the box: Everyday stories of death, bereavement and life*. PCCS Books.

Samuel, J. (2020). *This too shall pass: Stories of change, crisis and hopeful beginnings*. Penguin Life.

Samuel, J. (2022). *Every family has a story: How we inherit love and loss.* Penguin Life.

Van der Kolk, B. (2014). *The body keeps the score: Mind, brain and body in the transformation of trauma.* Penguin.

Wilson, J. (2020). *The plain guide to grief.* www.johnwilsononline.org

Audio/video

Munden, R. (2021). *Help.* Starring Jodie Comer and Stephen Graham. A Channel 4 drama about a care home worker and a resident with young onset Alzheimer's who form a bond – then Covid strikes. bit.ly/3AXe061

Rice, K. (2021). *Stolen goodbyes.* Personal stories of Covid-19 loss and grief. https://play.acast.com/s/stolen-goodbyes; www.audible.com/pd/Stolen-Goodbyes-Podcast/B08LMVSDTF; www.youtube.com/channel/UC_5XCNQClMzP3PIO5AjgrTQ (accessed 7 April 2022)

Samuel, J. (2021). *Soothe your pain, build your strength and heal.* Grief work app. https://griefworkscourse.com/?utm_source=js&utm_medium=website&utm_id=0

Selman L (2021) *Grieving during the COVID-19 pandemic.* www.youtube.com/watch?v=pi_11oq_nJg (accessed 7 April 2022)

Research/articles

Harrop, E. & Selman, L. (n.d.). *Bereavement during Covid-19: A national study of bereaved people's experiences and the impact on bereavement services.* An ongoing national study with several different foci. www.covidbereavement.com

Jackson, C. (2022). Navigating complex grief. *Therapy Today, 33*(6), 18–23.

Selman, L. (2021). Covid grief has cracked us open: How clinicians respond could reshape attitudes to bereavement – an essay. *British Medical Journal, 374*(1803).

Selman, L., Sowden, R. & Borgstrom, E. (2021). 'Saying goodbye' during the COVID-19 pandemic: A document analysis of online newspapers with implications for end of life care. *Palliative Medicine, 35,* 1277–1287.

Sowden R., Borgstrom E. & Selman L.E. (2021). 'It's like being in a war with an invisible enemy': A document analysis of bereavement due to COVID-19 in UK newspapers. *PLOS One,* 4 March. https://journals.plos.org/plosone/article?id=10.1371/journal.pone.0247904

Websites/online resources

At a Loss. Signposting website to help bereaved people find support, with some specific Covid support. *www.ataloss.org*

The Compassionate Friends. Supports bereaved parents and families when a child has died, irrespective of the child's age or cause of death. *www.tcf.org.uk*

Covid-19 Bereaved Families for Justice Group. *https://covidfamiliesforjustice.org*

Cruse Bereavement Services. National bereavement organisation providing telephone, online and face-to-face support. *www.cruse.org.uk*

Good Grief: A virtual festival of love and loss. Videos of events organised and hosted by the Good Grief Project. *https://goodgrieffest.com*

Good Grief Project. Organisation dedicated to understanding grieving as a creative and active process. *www.thegoodgriefproject.co.uk*

Health Talk. People talking on video about their own experiences of a huge range of health issues. Has a section on bereavement. *www.healthtalk.org*

The Hospice Biographers. Organisation that supports people to record their dying loved one's life story. *www.thehospicebiographers.com*

Hospice UK National organisation for hospice and palliative care. *www.hospiceuk.org*

Julia Samuel. Advice, support and resources about living with bereavement and stress. Includes information about her books and interactive app on the coping with grief. *https://juliasamuel.co.uk*

National Bereavement Alliance. Supports those who work with bereaved people. *www.nationalbereavementalliance.org.uk*

Samaritans. Suicide prevention helpline. *www.samaritans.org*

Silence of Suicide. Suicide prevention charity. *www.sossilenceofsuicide.org*

Yellow Hearts to Remember – COVID-19. Private Facebook group to remember people who have died during the pandemic. *www.facebook.com/groups/669274300301274*

York St John Bereavement Support Group. *www.yorksj.ac.uk/working-with-the-community/communities-centre/support*

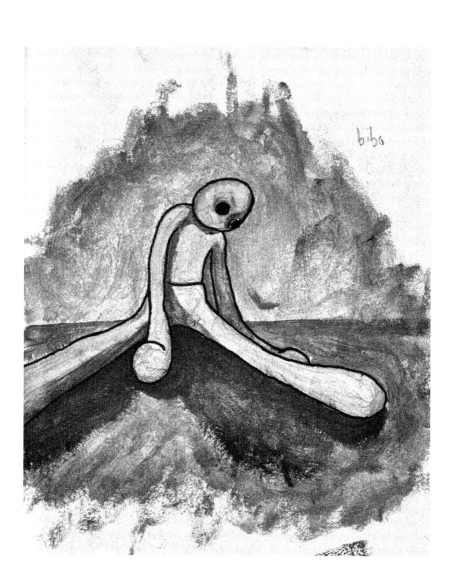

4.

Our future

Hello me

I got to know myself a lot better. To know what I like and don't like. Anything else? No. That's it.

The worry monster

I am nine and I kind of enjoyed lockdown. I didn't have to go in the car, and I get car sick so that was good. Daddy was teaching me because Mummy had to work full time from home. He checked my work every day. I did get bored, and I did not want to do the homework. I missed doing my swimming and gymnastics and seeing my friends, but I did do a lot of dancemat typing and now I don't just use two fingers anymore and I don't have to look at the keys. I was worried about my family getting sick. I write things down in my secret diary. It is very private. No one is allowed to see it, apart from the cover. I feel better when I have written things in there. And I got given a worry monster. It has rainbow fur and green hair and a zip on its mouth. You write down your worries and fold them up or screw them up and put them in there and they disappear. It lives on my bed and sometimes I cuddle it at night. It helps.

We got a dog

Tomos Price

When I think about lockdown, I think about my dog. We got her just before it all shut down. I had always wanted one. So I got to play with the dog a lot and take her for walks with my family. Brilliant! She's called Nala and she's lovely. I did do a lot more drawing because there was nothing else do apart from Xbox. I got quite good at it. I wasn't before. Otherwise, it was boring. I don't like being left to do my work myself. And now we have to do a lot of catching up. No one in my family got sick but our neighbours did. They were really ill but not with Covid. We were worried. They have always been kind to us. They give us apples and berries from their garden. They did get better.

My birthday was in lockdown, so we played Pictionary on Zoom and we ate all of the cake. We had a village group chat and one time we all played bingo. A man down the road has a big speaker and so we would call out the numbers and everyone would sit outside in their gardens and fill in their bingo cards. It was cool. Another time we did a quiz and we had drinks and food outside and we were all chatting at a distance. It was the first time I had played with any other children for ages. We went up and down on our bikes and had pizza. I missed my friends. It was so exciting when we saw each other again.

The coat

Katherine Brownlee, Service Director, Wiltshire Treehouse

When I met C she was sat anxiously in her seat wearing an oversized jacket. The classic, slightly tatty jacket didn't seem to match the other clothes of this teenage girl who had just joined our bereavement support programme. It was an odd addition to her outfit, but then again, we were all wearing layers of jumpers and coats as we tried to stay warm against the chilly winter air that was coming in through the windows that were open for ventilation (a hopeful safeguard against Covid-19).

During the course of the programme, this young person would sit (wrapped in the oversized jacket) and tell me about the overwhelming guilt she felt. She told me how she had caught Covid-19, and that her dad had then caught it from her. During one session, she tearfully relayed how the virus had struck him down, and that he had soon died in hospital.

She also spoke of her anger that she was not allowed to visit him in hospital due to visiting restrictions. She was angry that the chance to say sorry, and ultimately goodbye, was taken from her.

It wasn't until some weeks into the programme that she told me that the oversized jacket belonged to her father. She couldn't bear to be parted from it. Wearing it gave her a sense of comfort. It made her feel like she was close to him one more time.

The darkest period

Reflecting back on the darkest days of Covid lockdowns is quite a feat for me, as it was one of the most difficult periods I've ever encountered in my life, which is saying a lot since I'm only 16.

However, I think that highlights the severity of lockdowns on people's mental state, especially mine. I thought the first few weeks of the lockdowns were good as I secretly enjoyed the prospect of not needing to go to classes anymore and having all my exams switched online. But the weeks continued to drag on and I felt the loss of not having proper social interactions.

The joy I once felt slowly began to be overtaken by loneliness and feeling suffocated as my bedroom walls began to overwhelm and start to confine me. I began to realise the extent of how much I previously took simple things for granted – luxuries such as going to parties, outings, or even going shopping. I didn't view them as that until they were fully gone.

The things that I once considered as tedious at times turned into things I desperately craved as lockdown continued and the walls began to further creep in on me, pushing me further into confinement and despair. The days continued to go on and on and on… and eventually blurred together.

The motivation I felt once to speak to my friends and even my family began to decrease as time went on, and I felt myself being pulled into a deeper hole, which part of me felt I could never come back from. However, something inside me that I hadn't fully realised yet held onto something… *hope*.

Yes, as clichéd as it sounds, some part of me held on to something – a belief that I could make it out of this darkest of tunnels.

It's been more than a year since the last lockdown and it's been an uphill battle, but I can finally see the light that is beckoning me out of the darkest period in my life.

Home-schooled

I have been home-schooled since year 7 so in some ways my life stayed the same at home with my mum and dad and my sister. I have fewer ways of meeting people than you do at school anyway, and it definitely got worse under lockdown. No clubs, no sports. So sometimes I did feel a bit stuck. Just sitting in the same room at the same desk. It was hard to feel any kind of progress. At school, the goals are clear and you know if you are hitting them, and when you go up a year, your classrooms change, the activities change and you feel you are moving on.

At first, we did not really feel it was that serious. It was quite interesting. It didn't seem obvious Covid was a threat. No one close to us got really ill. So when the guidelines came out, it was sort of, 'Okay, well I guess we will do that.' Eventually we all had it, but we were lucky – none of us got really sick. Then it began to drag on. It was hard to get motivated to work.

At the same time, there were some real positives. I did more music and, because we could not go to church and I have done some video and editing before, I ended up responsible for all the livestreaming of services (my dad is the church pastor). It was really cool and great for my CV to show I have done that. We got loads of views from around the world, as well as from our church family in our town. I set up a YouTube channel and did all the editing. My skills really improved and I got really confident with it. And when you are less busy and taken out of normal life, it does make you think about what you really want to do. I guess 15 to 17 is always going to be a pretty formative period and maybe my confidence would anyway have been growing at that stage in my life.

We are a really tight-knit family, which significantly contributed to me coming out well from Covid. I can't imagine how I would have survived on my own, but I did begin to struggle with being with the same people for so long. I was lucky I could still get out and do my paper round and earn a bit of money. So many people lost their jobs.

I had a little period of about three or four months where it was really weird because I couldn't stop noticing my breathing. I was too self-aware and thinking about it all the time. I think I needed to go out and do some more normal stuff. I went out about a week ago with friends for first time in ages and we played pool. It was brilliant.

I never felt anxious about Covid. I am a Christian. I don't believe this life on earth is the end. I know I will go to heaven by the grace and love of Jesus.

Neurodiverse

Bill

I am a very indoor person. There is basically nothing I enjoy doing outside except walking the dog, which was still legal technically. Not sure what I did indoors. I don't really have an answer. It all blends together. I do spend most of my time indoors on computers. I like the computer world because it's malleable. Not as uncontrolled and random as outside. I did find doing schoolwork at home much harder and I did much less work, but I didn't miss school. Going back, I felt everyone was trying to hide how anxious they felt behind their masks. There really wasn't anything I didn't like about lockdown apart from worrying about my mum a bit, but she was sensible and took all the right precautions, so it wasn't too bad. I also worried about the effect on the economy and people's jobs, but it didn't really upset me.

Mum, I need help

Elizabeth Klyne

'Mum, I need help. Lots of help. I don't care for or about myself most of the time and I would like to. I feel really down. I would really like to be able to enjoy life.'

It's not the kind of message the parent of an 18-year-old longs to hear, but two years into our journey with PTSD, panic attacks and self-harm, this represented a massive step forward.

My son shut himself in his bedroom for a year between March 2020 and April 2021. He refused to come out or to speak. He rejected every single offer of love and support in whatever form we could think to bring it and hid under the bedclothes when I entered his room. He barely ate.

One day, I found bloodstains on the towels in the dirty washing basket. Then he appeared, like a wraith in black, rolled up his left sleeve and revealed a forearm etched with scars. My heart shattered into pieces.

At that moment, I wanted to rip out the creature inside him that had taken charge of my beautiful child's life – the entity that believed that inflicting pain was the only way to protect him from being overwhelmed by feelings that he did not have the capacity to process on his own.

Instead, I took a deep breath and welcomed the wisdom in him that had mobilised any way of keeping himself alive. I knew I was powerless in the face of this primal survival energy. Somehow, I found compassion for this destructive force within him and made peace with it. I thanked him for being willing to trust me.

Through days and months that stretched like mini lifetimes, I learned to resist the temptation to blame myself for everything he was going through. I waited and waited, holding a space of unconditional love and trust. My mind went on its own journey, but I didn't follow. Instead, I stayed present with this person who was insisting on the right to find his own way.

Then, in November 2021, a text out of the blue: 'I just realised that so many of the things I was doing aren't helping me at all. I just finally accepted who I am.'

My son had returned from his lonely journey into the darkness and was ready to accept support. My heart (which had sewn itself back together) leapt.

A deep appreciation

Lily Howard

My mental health hit rock bottom in the first lockdown, teaching me many lessons about myself and my outlook on life. The most valuable lesson was not the breathing exercises to combat the almost permanent panic attack but the importance of gratitude for what I do have.

In May 2021, I got a job as a waitress, simply to make some extra money for when I hoped to go to university. However, I never expected to gain such an invaluable perspective from working alongside some strong, beautiful people who help make up the diverse jigsaw that is the population of South London.

During my darkest nights, I could rely on my mum to hold me and tell me it was going to be okay, as she would never be further away than my living room. Then the next day I would head into work and hear my colleagues talk about how they hadn't seen their families for months and their trip home had been cancelled for the fourth time, due to Covid.

Our beautiful barista had not been able to see her mother since the pandemic began, yet never held a glimmer of resentment or jealousy when my mum would pop in for a coffee. She would greet her with a hug and kiss and tell her how she could tell she was an amazing mum, as she reminded her of her own mother.

I had the privilege of hearing stories from my workmates' home villages in Albania, Spain, Poland and Ukraine. Ordinary stories of people just trying to get on with their lives. Looking at pictures of Andalucia when my colleague came back from her long-awaited trip. The bliss radiated from her as she revelled in the fact that she got to take her dog for a walk again and bring back her favourite pair of boots that she left behind on her last trip in 2020. The joy she exuded brightened the hectic Saturday rushes, when we were all exhausted and covered in miscellaneous food and drink stains, reaffirming my faith in the power of family and love.

She showed me how devastating her separation was and is, as I had got lost in my own depression and struggles and hadn't stopped to consider how lucky I was to have my support system close to me.

We all counted down the days when someone booked a trip home, through each busy shift, until they could get on a flight, as no person deserved the separation my colleagues experience in those two years.

They became a second family to me and showed me that we all fought incredibly difficult individual battles during the pandemic, whether that was loss, loneliness or mental illness. Their strength and ability to keep laughing and bringing happiness to the people around them helped me to find light and small pieces of happiness again.

I realised that, if they could face such adversity, then we all can, by getting through each day and finding love and light in the smallest places. The lessons and wisdom they've given me are a debt I'll never be able to repay, and I feel privileged to know them.

To these colleagues I say thank you and tell you that I love you for all this.

I can't do the maths either

Emma

One positive was actually getting that period of time with your kids that you would not normally have. Got to really know them because you lose them when they go to school. They don't really tell you what they have been doing. One of the things that was unusual. Husband and I had split up before lockdown but were still living together. It was very artificial, but I was grateful we had not separated. Managing to have two separate spaces. Difficult if we meet someone else. Always was told could not work from home but have now done it for two years. Eldest nearly 12 and at secondary school. Matt, the little one, was 7. He did all the home-schooling. Hard to keep him on task, hard to focus, maybe on autistic spectrum. Once on it, then lazer focus. And eldest got on with it and I could continue working. Evie in year 6. She came to me for help with her maths. I had not got a clue. I did not even understand the question, and phoned a friend who is a primary schoolteacher. Mostly she got on independently. Felt a lot guilt. Too much telly. Not doing enough for your kids. We just have to get through this. Better with the summer and out in the garden. Got a large paddling pool. Ran up and down in the garden and bought a lot of fitness equipment. A real lifesaver. Got quite fit during lockdown.

Family in lockdown
Jackie Singer

Our family's version of lockdown was exacerbated by being in the middle of building works to our home, which were going on far longer than expected. Two adults and two young teens squashed into half a house with no kitchen, loud drilling, sometimes no running water or electricity was not much fun. We struggled, we shouted, we cried, doors were slammed. The teens lost confidence in dealing with people, became withdraw and anxious. Life was easier in their own bedrooms, online. We are still emerging from this, but one thing I will say: we have all got less attached to nice things happening. When Christmas 2021 was cancelled because of another bout of Covid, we pretty much all laughed it off. By then we had a house with no builders, a working cooker and a full fridge – bliss. As a parent, you never want your kids to experience trouble, but we do need it. It shapes our characters, and I think they are better off for not taking everything for granted.

Parenting in the pandemic
Nicky Hare

I have three children. One of them faced mock GCSEs in lockdown in the second lockdown; the others are younger. We live in a comfortable house; we have enough computers, and one school really rose to the occasion, offering a virtual online school day. We were actually quite excited the first time. A chance to all be together. We had to do it and so we settled in together, each of the children and my husband finding a workspace, getting themselves organised. My daughter put up a special shelf for all her workbooks. A bit of an adventure, despite the fear creeping around it all. We worried about the lack of food in the house until we got it sorted.

Soon, though, I began to feel like a hostage, creeping around all of them, having to be quiet, provide meals when needed (not always at the same time), prevented from having my own space and only able to get out with the dog once a day and occasionally meet other dogwalkers. I could not run (which is my passion) at first but I made sure I and the whole family were outside every single day. We live near a really good park, which made a huge difference. At first, we walked together; then the children started going off on their own, but at least we were out of the house. Then my daughter's school thought the children needed less screen time and asked parents to do some of the teaching with materials they sent over. My daughter and I found the assignments very boring and neither of us wanted to do them. Gradually it all got harder. My daughter started sleeping badly, not wanting to eat, really missing her friends and flying off the handle at the slightest thing. Just going into meltdown. The boys found it hard to keep engaged in lessons. Many pupils turned off their cameras so there was little sense of connection and so hard for the teachers, talking into a void. And we are the lucky ones in so many ways.

Tickets please

Richard Benwell

'Tickets, please' – for years, the main human contact at commuter o'clock, on the early train to London and the late train back. Of course, there were smiles and greetings, especially with the regulars on the Didcot to Paddington line, but the experience could be a hollow one.

Fast forward to 2020/21 and, for me, 'tickets please' is still a regular refrain in the morning. Now, though, it isn't from GWR livery, it's from the bright uniform of infancy. The request isn't droned, it's declaimed! The vehicle isn't the train, it's an ever-exciting and unquenchably magical imaginary bus. My son, Robin, loves to pretend that the top of the stairs is a double-decker and to invite passengers to join him to celebrate the wheels on the bus faithfully revolving. And, thanks to lockdown, I have a season ticket.

Before I go any further, I know very well that I'm one of the lucky ones. Coronavirus is a terrible affliction and the (very necessary) lockdowns brought untold unhappiness and hardship to so many people. Cruelly, they were often the people who were already in most need or most vulnerable.

But this story is one of reclaimed happiness and opportunity and I hope it's worth the telling for the reminder it gives us. Many millions of people have always made plenty of space in life for family, but there's no doubt that many millions of hours were also spent in unnecessary (and often unsustainable) journeys backwards and forwards. Many fathers and mothers missed out on golden hours of their children's young years because of work.

Instead of leaving the house before light and returning after bedtime several days a week, I've had the privilege of being at home so much more in the last couple of years. As restrictions lift, my colleagues and I have found a new normal where we can meet regularly enough to do good work, without squandering valuable time.

The unexpected gift of the pandemic has been that, instead of those monotonous journeys and long office hours, I've had the joy of almost every meal with family, and never missing the bedtime story. Watercooler moments in the office have been replaced with an impromptu daddy dance round the kitchen. Robin is definitely the boss.

One of the regular phrases people use to describe the disorientating and confusing changes Covid brought has been 'the world has gone mad'. But perhaps the Mad World was the one before, where we'd locked ourselves into routines that were unhealthy and unfulfilling. If we can salvage some good from this dreadful episode, perhaps it can be this: let's not fill up our lives again with too much that's unnecessary. The journey of life is too short. So let's take the more magical routes wherever we can. Tickets, please!

My Covid-19 autobiography

It all began when the rumours of a new virus spread. I didn't believe it at first and ignored it. Then the news began saying, 'The new virus Covid-19 has killed 100 people.' Still, I ignored it, and life was the same. Then the news got serious. It began to start saying thousands, and then I was scared. I'd go to school normally, but I was scared and told people 'A new virus is coming.' They had checked and were also scared. As I'd come home, they would say, 'Higher infection and death rate, might start new mask rule.' I said to myself, 'What's happened to life? Is this truly the end?' I would go to sleep, with the next day being death, death, death. It wouldn't stop, 10 thousand. 100 thousand. Millions, billions! As my final months of year 6 started, a test called the SATS was cancelled, and we were all happy.

Then it was Year 7. Corona destroyed my year 7 learning. Year 8 is like doing year 7 again as last year all we did was online learning. It was just, 'Students, here's your work.' Not much help, and connection problems also annoyed us. Lockdown began, life destroyed. I couldn't do much except sleep, online learning, repeat. That was life. Just again and again and again.

When eventually, the lockdown started to cool down, we went back to school. Soon after, positive and home again. I basically missed half the actual school year because of Corona. When I went back, I had to wear masks and things; it was so annoying and, since I have glasses, it steamed them up. They were very hot too. Sometimes they would make us wear masks outside. We missed the New Year party twice, and I was bummed about that. I also remember the NHS clap and people refusing to wear masks.

The year zoomed past and it's year 8 now. Everything's pretty good and the lessons are back to normal. I can go to my friends' houses and to the parks again; I can go to the cinema; everything is like Covid never happened, but a mild flu is just around. But I will never forget Covid. Covid killed my father's cousin. He was only 50. My dad works in a care home and during the first three months he came home saying 25 people died. His life was hard because so many people who he knew died. Earth was as if no one was on the planet. It was like humans were extinct. The weather had changed to sunny as there was no one to pollute.

Things didn't turn out the way I expected

Rhys Wathen

Covid came when I was in year 11 – towards the very end. At first, we all thought it was just like a bit of a cold. We really underestimated it. Next thing we knew, we couldn't even take our GCSEs. That was a big shock, and then they said they would be taking our grades from our mocks. Everyone was really stressed because none of us gave 100% in the mocks, apart from the last one we took after we knew. We worried about our future. Then came the first lockdown. Being cooped up in our houses. Everyone home 24/7 caused a lot of arguments. We had to adapt. We coped. Still could watch church every Sunday. That was good. It was hard not being able to see my mates. Lucky to have technology but it's just not the same. Could only get outside when I went for a run. Breaking up for summer in year 11 is supposed to be your time to do what you want. We didn't get that, or our prom. Only year in the history of the school not to have one.

I lost a bit of confidence about being social purely because of what Covid does to you. But you get used to it. Been pretty lucky, to be fair; no one I know has been really ill. So, I finished college in June and did a plumbing apprenticeship. That was messed up because of Covid too. I was on a one-year intensive course because I did okay with my grades but then, midway, there was a three-month lockdown. That had a big impact on us students. We had a big module to cover and no practical or theory stuff being taught. It was such a big wake-up call. Just had to go straight for it. Smash out everything. Get as much done as we could.

I did manage to finish the course and then I started looking for work. People kept saying, 'We read your CV and you would be an ideal apprentice, but we don't feel able to take anyone on because of the Covid situation.' I got it, but I needed a job. So I tried the bigger firms and I got lucky. This woman said, 'Yes, we are taking people on.' Got an interview. The guy interviewing me supports the same football team, so I was in! It felt brilliant. Honestly, best decision I have ever made. There was a lot of stuff going on in Swindon. A war between different territories – between gangs. Now I have no time for any of that. I am concentrating on getting my qualifications and working 60 hours a week. I'm earning, the job is fantastic and I am learning so much. I work with a great bunch of lads.

University life

I had just finished my second term of university in York when Covid started feeling real and restrictions were beginning to be announced. I remember my last night out in mid-March when the DJ shouted, 'Make some noise if you know who you want to self-isolate with!' At the time it felt like a joke. I came home from university with a small suitcase, convinced I would be returning for summer term in a few weeks. I wasn't able to return until June, when I travelled up for a day to collect my belongings. All my summer modules and exams were cancelled, so I was faced with an indefinite period of having absolutely nothing to do in my family home. This was simultaneously freeing and daunting. During the first lockdown, I taught myself saxophone, learned how to code, read a lot and started running.

At the start of the next academic year, I moved into my first student house in York, with six others. All my lectures and seminars during this time were online, which gave us an opportunity to spend lots of quality time together in the house. We would eat together, study together and we eventually started having party nights every Friday, where each of our rooms was a different 'club room', with its own theme. One way the pandemic affected me positively was academically: as well as being able to commit more time to studying, all my exams were open book and 24 hours long! Despite this, throughout second year, all my society activities were on Zoom or online; I was unable to continue playing in the orchestra and didn't meet many new people at all.

I am now currently living in Leeds for my final year and things feel very much back to normal. I have had many opportunities to connect and reconnect with people and all my lectures and seminars are now in person. Overall, while the pandemic dominated the majority of my university experience (I graduate in a few months), I am still very grateful for all the experiences I have had throughout it. I was 19 when it began and I am turning 22 this year, so it has contributed to a long period of my development as a young adult.

Struggling to adjust
Tom Grant Edwards, café worker

I was 18 when the first lockdown came. I had been working for a year, between four and six days a week in a café, and living at home. Suddenly, it all came to a stop. At first it was a bit of relief, like a holiday. I didn't have to get up and I was on furlough; less money but I did not have many bills to pay, so I was lucky. Then, after about a month, it began to get tedious. I had taken work for granted – the structure it gave me and all the interactions with people. When you are a barista, it is more than making a latte; it is all about those little conversations that can brighten up the day. I really began to miss work and I felt guilty about the money. It didn't really feel like mine.

I am really into my fitness, so I decided to spend money on building up a gym in our garden. I went on runs, weight trained and started to really study nutrition. I want to become a personal trainer. I started listening to my body and what I was eating and drinking, which felt good. Then, when we started to come out of lockdown, I found I was really anxious about being in large groups of people. I had begun selling clothes online and I didn't even want to go to the post office with my parcels. It was okay meeting a friend for a walk but going into a pub felt really difficult. It never happened at the gym. I guess I was just so focused on my goals there. I am still struggling with this. Like coming back to a reality I am not quite adjusted to any more. I don't feel there is much help out there with this sort of thing. You just have to try and work it out for yourself.

No one to turn to
Nate Thompson

I think when it did hit us all that those who were already struggling with mental health, depression, anything – it made it worse for everyone, but especially for those who were already struggling and now with Covid, it was much harder to reach out for the help they might've really needed. Since maybe before Covid was around it could've taken quite some time, but now it could take even longer for those who have been struggling longer too to reach out to the professionals for help and have regular meetings to check in with them and see how they're doing, especially with everything going on in the world. I know some of my own friends have had serious challenges with mental health and depression and I've always put them before myself so they can have the help they need and the support they need from others.

I reckon Covid showcased that, even with the plethora of things I might've done day to day after online school or during the breaks, I knew they were subtle distractions from the world outside and weren't going to be enough to properly distract me from the waves of depression that then led onto the mood swings I had, both during the first months of Covid and now, even when things seem to be going back to normal. It definitely still all affects me to this day, since I could suddenly be committed to something and then, just like that, it'll change, and I'll probably go back to it later or maybe even just not at all since I'll just forget about it and think nothing of it for some time.

I can also say that, with everything going on outside with the world, I definitely spent much more time in my room, since it felt like my own little comfort bubble; like a safe zone of just me, myself and I. Sometimes I wished for it all to be over, since it meant pushing back plan after plan. Like meeting a friend in person for the first time ever that was planned for the year Covid hit, but since then we have managed to meet. I'm glad. It was one of the best experiences in the past few years, since the friendship began as just strangers who had met on a livestream and now it's a sibling connection and I couldn't ask for a better older sibling than them since they mean the absolute world to me, and I would never stop putting them before myself since they deserve the whole world.

Rise in suicides
Lucy Coulbert, Oxford funeral director

What people weren't really thinking of or expecting throughout lockdowns and the ever-increasing Covid death rate was the amount of young people who weren't supported and then went on to die by suicide. In one particular month, all of the funerals we arranged and attended were for people who were under the age of 25.

Home learning
Alice Matthews, teacher

Online learning – some kids really thrived from it. One girl who is mute electively really started communicating through the chat function during online lessons. I was finally able to hear her thoughts. So the school have taken this on board and are aiming to continue to facilitate this. Equally, some quite cheeky boys in my year 10 class thrived off being at home alone. Not keeping up with their mates and instead they actually learnt because really they are intelligent and want to work. When I said I was surprised they said 'No miss. It is far more interesting to listen to you than do other stuff.' Quite a compliment really!

What has been really noticeable is that all my students find it really hard to plan long-term. Things have changed so much in the last two years, they cannot think beyond next week. It's hard to inspire and encourage aspiration. They cannot see that what they are doing now might impact their future. They just don't see how it all adds up.

A rather cocky year 7

I can remember coming back into school once a month to be with key workers' children and feeling so sorry for them. Not at home with parents, which for some was precious, and without distractions so aware of the frightening things their parents were going through. They missed their friends, and their friends were still doing online lessons. Interestingly, because they were in a small, all-age group, they mixed in well together. There are not many inter-year relationships usually. That was nice to see. Then they lost them again as they got put into year-group bubbles. The natural school hierarchy also disappeared with the year bubbles. Year 7 are usually intimidated by year 11 when they come up to secondary school, but this did not happen, so we had a rather cocky year 7!

Year 1

Sally Hinchliff, teacher educator

A bright morning in November 2021 and I arrived outside a small infant school, hidden away amongst myriad terraced streets. The school was close to the hills and near to a major city, but you would not have known it.

Due to the Covid-19 pandemic, it had been nearly two full years since I had set foot in a 'real' classroom. Instead, like many others involved in teacher education, I had embraced the 'new normal' of meeting my student teachers and their mentors via Zoom. So now, permitted again to go into school, I was so glad to return. This was a lovely place, with its own forest school, large playing fields and even a couple of goats. Recalling my last visit, I remembered the teachers as being kind and skilled and that the children seemed happy. Without a doubt, I had missed this school and many others like it: the hubbub of the classroom, the shouts and screams from the playground, the rows of small coats and piles of colourful lunch boxes and, perhaps most precious of all, the sight of small children sitting cross-legged on the carpet, listening attentively to their nervous student teacher as she told them a story (but then, who wouldn't be nervous with their university tutor sitting at the back of the room?).

Even as I entered the year 1 classroom where the student I'd come to observe was making the final preparations for his phonics lesson, I was aware of a nervous energy starting to pulse through my body. I put this down to the novelty of being back in a classroom, but as the lesson commenced, I felt increasingly uneasy. What hit me first were the absences. Where had the tables gone? Where was the reading corner with the comfy cushions? The carpet for telling the stories, discussing the maths problem and talking to your partner seemed to have disappeared altogether. Disorientated, I looked around me, trying to comprehend how a space so familiar – I might even say, a space I *loved* – had suddenly become alien and unrecognisable.

Then it dawned on me. It was the sight of a class of four- and five-year-olds trapped in tightly packed rows of desks that had triggered this almost visceral reaction. I struggled to focus on the student teacher, who was oblivious to his tutor's distress and forged on with the drill of 'segmenting' and 'blending' the phonics. Instead, I turned to the class teacher sitting beside me: 'It all looks so *different*?' was the only way I could think to articulate my confusion. In response she shook her head, paused, and then replied, 'It's our Covid catch-up curriculum... it has to be like this now, they are all just so far behind.' I wanted to bombard her with so many questions: 'Is this why none of the children leave their seats? Where has the carpet gone? Do they still have a story?' However, I asked none of them, aware that, once the floodgates opened, I might not be able to stop. Perhaps sensing my unease, almost inaudibly she said, 'It makes me so sad.'

Back in my car, out of sight of my student teacher and the school staff, I burst into angry, desperate tears. At the time, I was taken aback by how profoundly I was affected by a routine observation visit, but I understand those emotions better now. Many of us in education had hoped that, for all its horror, the Covid-19 pandemic might have ushered in a more relational, collaborative and creative form of schooling. The enforced isolation of the lockdown showed us how crucial a role school plays in the social world and, naïvely perhaps, I had expected change for the good. Instead, what I saw was a mean, limited and stifling classroom. I do not want this for any five-year-old, let alone those who have spent most of their young lives with the deprivations of the pandemic. So, in a way, I think I was crying for those children.

The wellbeing warriors

Diane Pummell, trainee child counsellor

I'm a trainee counsellor who uses art in my work, just completing my diploma in child counselling. I work at a large primary school in Twickenham – about 700–750 pupils on three sites. I was off work with Covid myself for 18 months, and when I went back into school, I noticed a big change in the atmosphere. I used to work with a lot of angry children. Now I wasn't seeing anyone for anger issues. I was curious about that. I also run the school council, where I have the opportunity to hear the children's voices. It's good for keeping me in touch with what they are thinking and needing. A lot were talking now about wanting a quiet space in school. There is a quiet area in the playground, but it's noisy; the kids run through it. Another need they talked about was to do more art, more creative things, outside the curriculum. And I thought, I'd love to create a therapeutic space in the school, a quiet area, where I could hopefully start to meet some of these needs. Quite rightly, the teachers and head want children out of doors at break time, but this expressed need wouldn't go away.

So, with the head teacher's support, I set up a club called Wellbeing Warriors – a Monday lunchtime drop-in club open to anybody in years 4 to 6. I was also aware that there's never enough of me to go round. I saw this as an early intervention – a quiet, safe, creative space where children can chat and things may come up that I can pick up early on.

In the first week, 13 came; by the third week it had grown to more than 30 – all girls. I didn't announce it; it just grew organically. We discuss topics like self-care and feelings, and a peer support culture is beginning to emerge. They are making new friendships and several children are finding their voice by talking about worries or sharing their experiences. I think the draw of football may be too strong for the boys to resist, although I am thinking about what a similar safe space for them might be.

When I ask the girls what they get from coming, they say things like, 'When I come here and just do art and I don't have to pick a topic and I can do it freely, I feel better and more able to cope with the afternoon in school'; 'I don't have many friends. Coming here helps me with that. I can have some time out and I feel better about the afternoon'; 'My aunt died of cancer recently, my whole family are sad, I draw colourful pictures and it helps me', and 'I often quickly went from feeling angry to sad, but now I seem to know how to handle things much better.'

They are valuing the calm, the freedom to express themselves. With no guidance from me, they are drawing sunsets and posters with words like Peace and Be Kind, and lovely creative images. Art is helping them to express their feelings. There's lot of splatting and sploshing with the brushes and sometimes little groups come in together and want to sit together and create images together, which has been lovely to observe.

Anxiety is still one of the main reasons I see children individually, but it's not big angry stuff now – more gentle talking about their horrible experiences during the pandemic and how it has left them with all these worries. The Wellbeing Warriors group meets a heartfelt need to have this downtime, this space for themselves. They sit pretty much in silence; there's sometimes a little whisper here and there. And it's just evolved this way. I haven't had to make it happen.

Commentary
Jo Holmes

Working as a school counsellor in a busy secondary school, pre-Covid, I was already well acquainted with the rising need for mental health support. Issues focusing on family relationships, fractured friendships, loneliness, loss, gender identity, body image and low self-worth were all common themes. As was childhood trauma in its widest context.

Mental health issues, including psychological distress, can present in a number of ways – from heightened anxiety to panic attacks, low mood, mood dysregulation, suicidal thoughts, disorderly eating and/or other self-harming behaviours. Some children may become withdrawn, disengaged, or just go under the radar, perhaps remaining hidden in plain sight. Some ask for help loudly, others have little or no voice.

As a result of the global pandemic, not only were children and young people with pre-existing mental health needs finding it hard; we also had a new generation of youngsters struggling. This was linked to changes in routine, unexpected challenges or feelings of isolation that came with being disconnected with life as we all once knew it and, of course, loss. We entered into unprecedented territory.

So how has it been for children and young people and how has their mental health fared during the pandemic? What can we learn from the stories these writers tell us in these moving accounts? What impact has there been on family life?

Rhys talks of the worries caused by cancelled GCSEs (p.113), which resonates with many similar stories from young people in their final year at school. He captures a sense of pure shock and disbelief linked to all his previous experience of education, acknowledging that he hadn't put his 'all' into his mocks and was alarmed that his grades were being taken from past papers. He worried about his future but, despite significant challenges, found himself an apprenticeship. He was determined and driven – his story is one of true resilience. But Rhys also tells us that his confidence wavered at times under the stress felt by his whole year group.

In her article in *The Telegraph*, Christina Hopkinson (2022) considers the distress caused to students linked to uncertainties about new Covid variants affecting the future of exams and testing children. One parent talks of her daughter's 'crippling panic attacks', describing these as 'her default response to testing'. While exams stopped, constant testing had become the Covid norm. On the one hand, there was a sense of relief from some young people that exams had been cancelled, but then came the pressure of how to grade student learning and, of course, coping with such massive change.

Loss and change were key themes throughout the various lockdowns. Jackie Singer writes of her family's experience during this time (p.110): 'The teens lost confidence in dealing with people, became withdrawn and anxious. Life was easier in their own bedrooms, online.' She goes on to talk about the resilience the family gathered along the way and learning not to take anything for granted. A wonderful insight into family togetherness and growth from that period.

Each family has their own unique experience but there were common themes captured throughout. Nicky Hare (p.110) shares the importance of being outside and walking through the park, and the contrast of her daughter beginning to struggle over time with eating, sleeping and having 'meltdowns'. These key mental health struggles, common before the various lockdowns, are now continuously described as issues 'exacerbated by the pandemic'.

A study published in *The Lancet* (Solmi et al., 2021) found that both urgent and routine referrals to specialist eating disorder clinics in the first year of the pandemic doubled from the previous year. Factors contributing to spikes in referrals ranged from social isolation to food insecurity, pressure to exercise, loss of routines and the impact of disruptions to accessing services.

We know there has been immense pressure on mental health services as a result of the pandemic. According to NHS Digital (2020), this has worsened since 2017, with one in six children aged 5 to 16 having a 'probable mental health disorder' – a rise from one in nine prior to the pandemic. The study also reported that 54% of young people aged 11–16 experiencing poor mental health said that lockdown had made their life worse, compared with 39% of those deemed 'unlikely' to have a mental disorder.

These findings are stark but not surprising. Buttle UK, in a series of podcasts (2021a) focusing on child welfare and poverty, discuss how the pandemic impacted on mental health. The message is clear: the pandemic has exacerbated (that word again) worries and anxieties for children and families alike, and for those families who experienced an increase in 'adverse childhood experiences', or ACEs, this was (and remains) of great concern.

The *State of Child Poverty 2021* report, also published by Buttle UK (2021b), found that low-income families were more impacted by the pandemic than more affluent counterparts. When asked to provide details on ACEs (the family situational factors that impact on child development and life chances), the most commonly reported themes were mental health problems, parental separation and domestic abuse, criminal exploitation and child sexual exploitation. A report published by the NSPCC (2020) found that the pandemic increased stressors on parents and carers, resulting in higher risks associated with child abuse at a time when there were fewer 'normal' protective services available. Children also had heightened vulnerabilities to other types of abuse, including online abuse, criminal exploitation and child sexual exploitation.

How do children and young people deal with these multiple and often traumatic experiences? How do they regulate emotions and worries? When anxieties become heightened, children may go into panic mode, due to the level of fear they experience, resulting in possible panic attacks. This can be in response to perceived threat or real fear linked to danger. We often talk of flight, freeze or flight. Young Minds provides excellent resources describing anxieties, panic attacks and how best to manage them (see the Resources section below). The resources can help families respond in the best way too.

We also know there has been an increase in reported self-harming behaviours and eating disorders, a rise in suicidal ideation (thinking about not wanting to live any more) and a rise in reported low mood.

The mother's breathtaking account of her 18-year-old son's experience of locking himself into his bedroom for a year, not talking, hardly eating, having panic attacks and struggling with post-traumatic stress disorder provides us with a glimpse of how difficult it was for some young people who were already struggling with their mental health pre-pandemic (p.107). She describes dealing with a force of 'primal survival energy' – her son was staying alive by cutting himself and inflicting pain. She understood that this was the only way he felt he could protect himself from being overwhelmed by his feelings. He simply didn't have the capacity to process any of his trauma on his own. The story is one of unconditional parental love. When her son was ready, he asked for help, but until he reached out and wanted some sort of change for himself, all his mum could do was keep him as safe as possible, while holding at bay her own feelings of guilt, despair and all those other things with which we beat ourselves up as parents. It's a story of survival.

The funeral director's account of the perceived rise in young suicides is poignant (p.117). So too is the story of the young woman wearing her father's jacket (p.104), full of unresolved guilt because he caught Covid from her and it killed him and she didn't have a chance to say sorry. There are several national and local charities that support children who have been bereaved of a parent or sibling. Details of some of them are in the Resources section at the end of this chapter.

It has been, and continues to be, a tough time for many children and families, and of course, not just those affected by trauma or a mixture of adverse childhood experiences. Any child from any background can be affected by poor mental health.

Despite this, NHS digital figures indicate how it isn't a level playing field and that some children and young people are more vulnerable to mental health struggles than others. For example, 63% of 11–16-year-old girls with a mental health diagnosis have seen or heard an argument between adults in their household, compared with 46% who were unlikely to have a 'mental disorder'. Added to this, children aged 5–16 years experiencing poor mental health are more than twice as likely to live in a household that has fallen behind with payments (16%) than children unlikely to have a mental disorder (6%).

Financial constraints are a crippling worry for many families. It's not much mentioned here but Gordon Knott's account of his work for the Croydon Drop-in Centre in Chapter 2 (p.53) paints a very vivid picture where he reminds us of the need for food banks during the pandemic. These are the stories that often go unheard. Online learning was practically impossible for many families unable to afford laptops and crammed into tiny flats where the children had no quiet space for study. Then there are the young people living with long Covid who describe in this chapter their struggles to keep up with schoolwork and maintain friendships .

Others reflect on the pandemic as a period in their lives where loneliness and feeling suffocated by bedroom walls was all consuming (p.105). Lily, who'd 'hit rock bottom', describes the joy she gained from securing a part time waitressing job and the connections she then made with her colleagues (p.108). There's no doubt that this period of normality, before going to university, was a huge boost for her. Many others continue to struggle with the loss of confidence and social skills described frequently here.

The pandemic was a time of uncertainty – so many plans were cancelled; so many expectations turned out not to be possible, as Rhys describes (p.113). Some will have developed emotional resilience, others will continue to struggle, and many of these struggles may remain hidden for years to come.

But there are positive stories too. We know some children and young people who, like Bill (p.107) and Nate (p.116), perhaps because they are neurodiverse, benefitted from the changes, and from being sanctioned to spend more time and study on their own at home. The mandatory rules and regulations made their lives easier. The teacher's description of a child who had lost her voice through elective mutism and who was able to thrive by using the chat function of online learning is a wonderful account (p.117), and also to know that the school now realised the potential here for children who feel less able to be vocal in class. It's also heart-warming to read about trainee counsellor Diane

Pummell's successful venture to create a safe space within her school to meet the pupils' need for a quiet, contemplative place where they can make art and just be together (p.120).

Without wanting to invalidate the many struggles families experienced during this period, we must acknowledge that, for some, it was also an opportunity to spend more time together, learn new skills and become more resilient in exceptionally difficult circumstances. There's no doubt that access to outside green space also helped with this.

Alongside an appreciation for nature, the accounts in this chapter offer some insightful ways of managing distress – from the nine-year-old who talks frankly of the comfort gained from her 'worry monster' and writing things down (p.103) to neurodiverse Bill (p.107) who enjoyed going outside to walk his dog. These small, everyday activities help, regardless of the circumstances.

Sometimes we need additional help too. Children and young people need to be listened to, to talk openly about their worries and to own them. If a child tells an adult they are sad or they are struggling, we need to hear what they are saying, and not always jump straight into trying to make it better for them. Rather than attempt to rescue them, we need first to respond with validation – 'That sounds tough' – and then ask them to think about what kind of things may help.

We perhaps won't know for years to come the real long-term impact of the Covid years on children and young people's mental health and what they missed out on at such a critical time in their development. What we can do is support them through it and help them draw on their own resources and the wide range of support out there for them.

References

Buttle UK. (2021a). *All in the same boat? Inequality, children and their future. Greg Rutherford learns about children and their mental health.* Podcast. https://buttleuk.org/news/all-in-the-same-boat

Buttle UK. (2021b). *State of child poverty 2021.* Buttle UK. https://buttleuk.org/news/news-list/state-of-child-poverty-2021

Hopkinson, C. (2022, January 25). Are we testing our children too much? *Daily Telegraph.* www.telegraph.co.uk/education-and-careers/2022/01/25/testing-children-much

NHS Digital. (2020). *Mental health of children and young people in England, 2020: Wave 1 follow-up to the 2017 survey.* https://digital.nhs.uk/data-and-information/publications/statistical/mental-health-of-children-and-young-people-in-england/2020-wave-1-follow-up#

NSPCC. (2020). *Social isolation and the risk of child abuse during and after the coronavirus pandemic.* NSPCC Learning. https://learning.nspcc.org.uk/research-resources/2020/social-isolation-risk-child-abuse-during-and-after-coronavirus-pandemic

Solmi, F., Downs, J.L. & Nicholls, D.E. (2021). Covid-19 and eating disorders in young people. *The Lancet: Child and Adolescent Health, 5*(5), 316–318. www.thelancet.com/journals/lanchi/article/PIIS2352-4642(21)00094-8/fulltext

Jo Holmes is the Children, young people and families lead at BACP (British Association for Counselling and Psychotherapy), based within the policy team, and is a qualified person-centred counsellor. Jo has a background in youth work and has worked in a full range of settings, leading on health education projects, including sexual health and drugs work. Jo worked on the extended schools agenda, based within a family of schools, eventually retraining as a counsellor as she was finding increasingly that her work involved supporting children and young people who were struggling with their mental health. Having experienced the benefits of offering early-help counselling intervention in schools, but with no additional funding, Jo now advocates for universal access to government-funded counselling in schools, colleges and wider community settings across England (in line with the rest of the UK). *www.bacp.co.uk/news/campaigns/school-counselling*

Resources

Books

Abrams, R. (1992). *When parents die.* Charles Letts.

The Book Trust offers a reading list of books on bereavement and death for younger children. www.booktrust.org.uk/booklists/g/grief-and-loss-5-8-year-olds

You can find book lists for teenagers on bereavement and death at **www.thelisteningear.org.uk/young-people/books**

Websites/organisations

Action for Happiness. Daily online resources for positive and mindful activities for all ages and settings. *https://actionforhappiness.org*

BEAT Eating Disorders. Information, guidelines for good practice, helplines and web chat for people with eating disorders and their families. *www.beateatingdisorders.org.uk*

Carers Trust. Support and resources for carers, including young carers and young carers in schools. *https://carers.org*

The Charlie Waller Trust. Resources and support to help children, families, schools and other professionals look after their mental health. *https://charliewaller.org*

Child Bereavement UK. Supports children and young people (up to the age of 25) when someone important to them has died or is not expected to live, and parents and the wider family when a baby or child of any age dies or is dying. *www.childbereavementuk.org*

Childline. Free 24/7 confidential helpline, online chat and email for children. Tel: 0800 11 11. Children can request a free 1-2-1 chat at https://www.childline.org.uk/get-support/1-2-1-counsellor-chat/. A BSL interpreter is provided for deaf and hearing impaired children. *www.childline.org.uk*

Grief Encounter. Support for bereaved children and young people. *www.griefencounter.org.uk*

Harmless. Support for people to overcome self-harming and suicidal thoughts. *https://harmless.org.uk*

Hope Again. The youth website of Cruse Bereavement Support where they can learn from other young people how to cope with grief and feel less alone. *www.hopeagain.org.uk*

Mermaids. Free helpline, webchat or text 9am-9pm for young people and their families exploring gender. Tel: 0844 334 0550. *www.mermaidsuk.org.uk*

MindEd. Educational resource on children, young people, adults and older people's mental health with online learning platforms to help understand mental health issues and support young people. *www.minded.org.uk*

MindEd for Families. Families can access MindEd resources here. *https://mindedforfamilies.org.uk*

The Mix. Free helpline and support for anyone under 25, including free short term counselling, 1:2:1 webchat, email, crisis messenger. Tel: 0808 808 4994. *www.themix.org.uk*

Muslim Youth Helpline. Faith- and culturally sensitive support via free calls, live chat or email 4pm-10pm daily. Tel: 0808 808 2008. *https://myh.org.uk*

National Autistic Society. Advice, support and services, including information on mental health. *www.autism.org.uk/advice-and-guidance/topics/mental-health*

Reading Well. National organisation promoting better health through recommended reading lists, with sections on mental health, children and young people, including self-help, personal accounts and information on common mental health challenges. Also accessible reading for 13–18 year olds. All available at local libraries in England and Wales. *https://reading-well.org.uk/books/books-on-prescription*

Samaritans. 24/7 free confidential helpline for whatever issue you need to bring. Tel: 116 123; email jo@samaritans.org. *www.samaritans.org*

SWGfL (South West Grid for Learning). Online safety training and other tools and resources to ensure children benefit from technology free from harm. *https://swgfl.org.uk*

TAC Access. 'Team Around the Child' linking professionals with commissioners to contract in qualified and competent counsellors and therapists who specialise in working with children and young people. *www.tacaccess.com*

Winston's Wish. Support for children, young people, families and professionals after the death of a parent or sibling (including when they took their own life). Free national helpline **08088 020 021** (9–5 Mon-Fri). *www.winstonswish.org*

Young Minds. National mental health charity with accessible online resources about mental health for children and young people and their families/carers and professionals. Free 24/7 text message service, text 85258. Helpline and webchat for parents/carers, tel: 0808 802 5544. *www.youngminds.org.uk*

Youth Access. Free and confidential counselling, advice and information services nationwide. *www.youthaccess.org.uk/services/find-your-local-service*

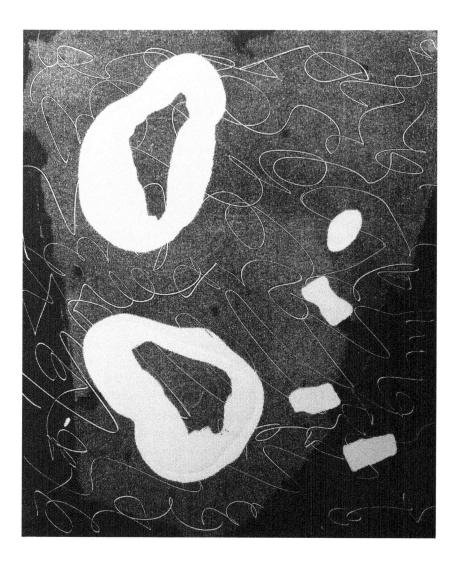

5.

Long Covid

Fatigue is not like tiredness

Unless someone has experienced it, it's hard to convey what the fatigue is like – one day, despite being incredibly thirsty all day, I remember not having the energy to reach for the glass of water on my bedside table until 2.00pm.

Living with long Covid

Claire Hastie

I am a single parent of three boys, and all of us caught Covid in Spring 2020. Luckily my 15-year-old was not seriously ill, because he had to do all the cooking and housework as I was bedridden for weeks. He roped in his 11-year-old twin brothers to help when they felt well enough, although they were also ill for months, and we all still experience relapses 15 months after falling ill. When I woke up with swollen glands a week before the first lockdown in March 2020, I erred on the side of caution and kept my children home from school. A few days later, my Mother's Day gift was feeling like I had been run over – I was short of breath, with what felt like an elephant sitting on my chest, frozen to the core and aching all over. I couldn't utter a sentence without gasping for air. As the symptoms worsened throughout the day, I knew I was seriously ill, so I forced myself to fire up my laptop to email colleagues to ask them to pick up my work (I'm a consultant and copywriter for a corporate reporting agency). The following weeks are a bit of a blur. When the weather was warm enough, I would drag myself out of bed into the garden, as it was easier to breathe outside. Lying on my front also helped, so I lay face down on a picnic rug all day, covered in blankets as I felt so frozen, unable to do anything except watch the bees buzzing about on the spring flowers. I couldn't read, watch TV or listen to the radio, as my brain felt overwhelmed with sensory overload. I went from cycling 13 miles a day on my commute to work to being unable to leave the house, and later only with the help of a wheelchair. Thankfully, although my kids had never been so ill, between their acute episodes of nose bleeds, sickness and diarrhoea, they generally were able to watch TV or play computer games, which is just as well, as I was too ill to care for them. My kids were left to their own devices – literally.

Over the first three months of being ill, I was advised five times, either by 111 or my GP, to go to A&E as my symptoms developed or worsened. Each time I was sent home, despite symptoms including tachycardia that lasted for hours, sharp pain in my lower lungs, heart pain, and severe pressure in my head accompanied by pins and needles and tinnitus. Perhaps oddly, the times when I felt worst, I was too ill to even call 999 or shout for my kids. More than once I was surprised to wake up the next morning. I spoke to one of my 11-year-old sons who happened to be passing my bedroom, telling him that if I didn't make it, I had had a great life and that he would be able to imagine what I might say or do in certain situations so I would haunt him that way! I thought best to keep it as light-hearted as possible for that type of conversation, as I didn't want to frighten him. If anything, it was the opposite – I have a vague recollection of having crawled up the stairs and collapsing at the top. He was babbling away to me about computer games while I fought unsuccessfully to stay conscious. I think he was completely oblivious to quite how ill I was – probably no bad thing.

I had done all the legal stuff – my will, who would look after the children, Lasting Powers of Attorney and the paperwork to donate my body to science – in my early 30s after having my first child. I had begun writing my end of life wishes (the 'softer stuff' about whether to resuscitate, who to contact and so on) after a family funeral a couple of years ago but hadn't got around to completing them.

I knew I had to finish them, as I'd heard how stressful it can be for grieving family members to have to second-guess what care their loved one wants in their final days, or their wishes for after death. Being too ill to read, I downloaded the audio version of Kathryn Mannix's book

With the End in Mind[1] so I could check I'd thought of everything. I was barely able to concentrate and kept falling asleep as I was so ill, but I eventually scraped together what little energy I had to complete my end-of-life wishes, which I shared with my mum and sister.

My kids and I are still living with long Covid, although we are hopeful of recovery – at least, enough to have a decent quality of life. I'd like to think I will no longer need the wheelchair at some point and be able to return to my job, after more than a year off. Having come so close to death, I am even more appreciative of the little things in life, and more mindful of how things can change in an instant. Life is precious, so I make sure I do what I love and spend time with people I love.

In my early weeks of being bedridden with Covid, I set up a Facebook group[2] to share information and support for those struggling to recover. The group now has now nearly 50,000 (February 2022) members in more than 100 countries and continues to grow. It is sad to see the numbers rising, but I'm also glad that people are finding us so we can support each other through what, for most of us, is the most challenging experience of our lives. Some of us have remained ill for 23 months and counting. But I do look forward to a day when the group no longer needs to exist – then we will have succeeded.

Energy begets energy (as long as you avoid burnout!)

I fell ill in March 2020 before the first lockdown. My commute to work was in a lift-share. One person entered the car with Covid, and an hour later five people left that car with Covid.

I made the decision to quarantine myself when I first started showing symptoms. I had headaches, terrible fatigue, stomach upsets, briefly a runny nose, but no cough and no temperature. But, after about a week of flu symptoms, I entirely lost my sense of taste and smell (this was before that symptom was recognised and reported as common). Then, a few days after that, I started struggling to breathe. I couldn't get a full deep breath, my breathing always felt shallow, like I couldn't reach the bottom of my lungs. It was hard to breath lying on my back, and it seemed to help if I lay on my front or my side. So I lay down for several days.

---

1. Mannix, K. (2022). *With the end in mind: How to live and die well.* William Collins.

2. www.facebook.com/groups/longcovid

I went from running 5km three times a week and hiking up mountains to not being able to walk up the stairs without lying down to get my breath back. I live alone. I was scared. At the height of the illness, I asked for a phone appointment with the doctor. I couldn't even speak a whole sentence in one go without stopping to breathe. The doctor, sadly, was patronising and unhelpful. I got the impression he thought I was exaggerating (for what purpose?!) and suggested we 'count my breaths together' as if talking to a five-year-old who just needed calming down. Eventually I told him (through struggling breaths), 'I've been managing this at home, and I am trying to keep myself out of the NHS equation. I'm an intelligent and educated woman. I just need to know at what stage I should seek extra help because after three weeks I'm still struggling to breathe, and I live alone.'

His answer: 'If your lips turn blue, call an ambulance.'

It was not long after talking to that doctor that my breathing started to improve and, luckily, my lips never did turn blue. I was still experiencing other symptoms. I had terrible fatigue, headaches and brain fog; I felt sore and achy, and I still couldn't smell anything nearly two months after my symptoms began. A friend would bring food shopping and leave it in the garden. There was still no clear guidance on how long contagion would last. So, for as long as I had some symptoms, I continued to quarantine myself and stay isolated. This lasted for nearly four months. By that time, I had found 'Long-haul Covid' groups online and felt reassured that I wasn't the only one.

I had a garden and tried to spend time in the sun to keep my vitamin D topped up. I focused on health and rest. And then, gradually, I began to increase my activity.

A walk round the block. Rest.

A walk a little further. Rest.

A five-minute jog around the block, walking if I needed to. Rest.

By late summer, I was starting to feel more like myself and was running and hiking again, but would still have occasional bouts of fatigue and brain fog. There were random days when I couldn't hang the washing on the line in one go. I'd do a couple of bits, then rest, then a couple more, then rest. This was even if I'd been able to run 5km the day before. There seemed to be no pattern to when it struck. And I've just had to learn to live with it and manage my energy levels carefully.

I still have occasional days when the fatigue will wipe me out and all I can do is stop and rest. If I plan to run and that day feel fatigue, I will rest. And run the next day. I treat my energy and time as a precious resource now, and I am careful to keep it balanced and not overdo it. I say no to things. I will not take on more than my energy will allow in a day (learning where that limit is can be part of the challenge!). I have found that, as long as it is increased gradually and I don't tip into burn-out, then energy begets energy. The more I do, the more I am able to do, gradually, over a period of time.

I always listen to my body. And if I find myself in the company of fatigue, I will rest with it, but I will not assume that I am ill all over again. Most days now there is energy, and if not today, then tomorrow.

Now, over two years down the line, I am training for a half marathon. I couldn't have believed that would ever be possible back then. I feel strong and I have energy (which I don't take for granted). This week I ran 10 miles (and felt great!), so my body seems to be on board and I'm confident I will achieve it.

A vicious cycle

I am one of the few men who is living with long Covid. I was getting more and more frustrated with myself as I did not understand why I couldn't seem to understand the simplest of things. Unbeknownst to me, at the time I was suffering with brain fog. I would repeatedly explain to my Head of Department that I was struggling both physically and mentally, yet was always reminded that a deadline was looming. I tried to explain what I struggled with, but felt I wasn't really being taken seriously. I was still not sleeping and the brain fog was worse the more tired I was.

It's really hard to explain the boom-bust cycle to friends, colleagues and family. This is not helped by the calcified government line that long Covid is a mild, flu-like illness. The lack of support led to outbursts of frustration, uncontrollable crying and depression, and I continued to experience a wide range of debilitating physical symptoms. It feels like a vicious cycle of being unwell with an illness no one properly understands, which means I don't recover properly because, as a teacher, it is impossible to adjust my working conditions. Teaching is unforgiving; if you're there, you give 100%, no excuses.

I had to learn to heal myself

Josie Webber

Calling 999 was very difficult as they kept asking more questions and I felt I couldn't breathe or get enough air. If I tried to stand up, my oxygen saturation levels kept dropping, and the vertigo and nausea were so acute I could only manage to stand for a minute or two. After the first six weeks of struggling, I bought myself an electric wheelchair in order to look after my two very active boys. Kidney infections, three in a row, made me very unwell in the first few months. And since then I've had chronic kidney pain. The doctors can't explain this.

Since getting Covid, I have become hypersensitive to noise. Even someone doing washing up in the room next door overloads my system if I'm having an energy crash. Visitors are very well intentioned, but the best ones don't talk much and sit very quietly when my energy dips, and are happy with companionable silences. I love it when friends and family visit and just get on with their own thing, in the same room. Joy! I love the presence of another adult in the house. For five months last year, my dear friend Denise moved over from the States to live with us and helped with cooking. She was awesome. The kids loved her.

I've had to learn how to have pre-emptive conversations before socialising, and my assertiveness skills need work. Covid is teaching me many things. My boys need my best listening and talking hours, and even they've had to learn to be quiet and use headphones or go outside to play football to allow me to have rest times. They've been extremely understanding and wonderful. Initially, my functional time standing or sitting up was so limited that I built up a huge pile of admin that needed attention and financially I was in a mess.

In her book, *Breaking Free: A guide to recovering from chronic fatigue syndrome and long Covid symptoms*,[3] Jan Rothney says that, similar to CFS and ME, feeling highly stressed for a number of years before getting Covid can make you more likely to get long Covid. I had been feeling for some years that life as a single parent was all too much, and that I'd had enough. I wanted some peace and extended time to myself, and some creative time. I certainly got that in the

---

3. Rothney, J. (2022). *Breaking free: A guide to recovering from chronic fatigue syndrome and long Covid symptoms*. Arkbound.

lockdown, and then with long Covid. What I've ended up with has been an enforced and very extended retreat, while still needing to parent and earn a wage.

I have found that a low histamine diet and antihistamines and supplements really made a difference to me. Sunlight also seems to help. Preferably several hours a day lying in the sun. Some say this is because, as well as giving the best vitamin D, sunshine is a powerful antiviral. Initially, resting wasn't really resting. I was fretting about what had happened to me and anxiously texting friends. Avoiding black tea and coffee and processed sugar and upping my seasonal organic fruit and veg consumption have been hugely helpful in reducing symptoms.

I stopped watching TV as it made me feel depressed and overwhelmed. After getting bogged down with others' Covid horror stories on some Facebook support groups, I discovered fellow long Covid sufferer Suzi Bolt's Facebook group, Yoga and Meditation for Gentle Covid Recovery.[4] It led to much more positive self-resourcing and I'm hugely grateful to her. The benefit of regular meditation/mindfulness has been huge to ease anxiety and help me feel more trusting of life. The increased calm has helped me to problem solve my way through this more easily.

I learned that if I managed to drop off during a rest three times a day, even for a few seconds, my system was more able to cope with being upright. This is still the case 20 months later. Without three rests a day, my symptoms still become really acute and frightening. Stress makes things a lot worse, so I am learning how to minimise it.

I have tried a number of treatments that others have found beneficial but some have had the opposite effect on me or simply not worked. For example, there is a theory that low levels of oestrogen might contribute, but HRT did not help me, whereas probiotics do. It seems each individual has to find their own healing pathway. My system is clearly still too reactive to cope with many treatments.

My main work is music teaching, and although I have cut my hours down by 75%, I still need to earn, being the only adult in my household. Teaching complex music or advanced theory is now out of the question. My memory and ability to find words and concentrate are so limited.

---

4. www.facebook.com/groups/1095053437543132

Even now, if I'm not very well rested, I get energy crashes during lessons where I can't hold my head up or speak or move my hands. It can be very hard to disguise that, so I have to time things carefully and be upfront with students so they are not alarmed. Performing can be precarious if an energy crash comes on during the gig.

I have had to learn to heal myself. In the first lockdown before getting ill, I started writing and recording a lot more of my own music. When I have an energy window and I can, this is the most healing medicine I have. The joy and connection to life in all its magic and mystery is alive and well then, and so am I.

This is not a game
Meredith Debonnaire

I have been spending a lot of time recently thinking about a (now obsolete) Flash Player video game, whose name I can no longer remember. Bear with me. In this game, you play as a virus. There's a map of the world, with animated planes and ships moving between the countries. As a player, your aim is to infect the entire world and kill as much of its population as possible – somewhat dark, but a fun, logistical challenge for a bored teenager. You use resources to change up the virus symptoms and how infectious the virus is. What is striking about this game is that it is nearly impossible to have a complete win, because the countries all shut down their airports and stop letting ships into their ports. Getting Iceland or Madagascar is near impossible.

I've been thinking about this game a lot. About the assumption of whoever coded this game that sensible, logistical decisions would be made about closing airports and limiting travel, and that, in the face of a terrifyingly infectious new disease, countries would have sensible isolating policies. I caught Covid in March 2020. About three days before, there was a national lockdown in the UK. I have not recovered. I am now 30, and I've been ill since I was 28.

I don't know how to talk about my personal experiences, and I almost don't want to. I am endlessly, ruthlessly, exhaustingly angry. Not just about the fact that I caught the illness, but that the things in place for someone with a chronic illness are so very difficult to access. At the time of writing, I am waiting to hear back about a Personal Independence Payment (PIP) application that I started making nearly six months ago. I have my first appointment with a Post-Covid Unit in a week, a year after I was referred. There has been very little accessible support available in the meantime: the underlying assumption appears to be that I live with someone who can pick up the slack caused by my illness. That I have access to a car. That I have access to a printer. That I have enough energy to read through the five different PDFs on self-care with fatigue that I have been sent. That I have enough energy to keep a fatigue diary. That I will remember what we have discussed and be capable of implementing it.

It does not help that I already have PTSD (which I do not have an official diagnosis for, because as far as I can tell there is one person in the UK who can do this and they are very busy and my GP doesn't know how to get me to them). Medical appointments trigger massive anxiety for me, so even getting myself to a doctor was already a mission when I had energy. I do not doubt that my GP is doing her absolute best, but the system set up around her requires that I am the one who does the chasing up if something is wrong. When the problem is that I have chronic fatigue and brain fog and chronic pain, this is devastatingly flawed as a system.

I am 30. I cannot do my own food shopping, because I cannot carry more than one bag at a time. I cannot do my own laundry because I cannot carry my washing to the launderette any more. If the air is cold, I cannot breathe properly. If I lie down wrong, the chest pain that I have had since March 2020 translates into my mind as a weight and sets off panic attacks that can last all night. This has led to the discovery that, yes, I can have insomnia *and* chronic fatigue. Joy.

I think about the stupid video game, and I think about how different any of this might be if the structures around us were different. I think about how long it took the UK to stop international travel and how early we reopened it. I think about the people on my high street who accost me to tell me that Covid is a hoax – the high street that I can no longer reliably walk up in one go because it is on a hill and I cannot walk up hills. I had a roaming range of about 10 miles before I was ill, and that was with a cartilage-damaged knee. I am excited these days if I can walk two miles, and I use a cane because I am too fatigued to do the physiotherapy that keeps my knee healthy enough to walk on it.

I have accepted that this is a new condition, and that no one can tell me what will happen or whether I will get better. I cannot accept that there is no help for me now. If this is my new normal, I need help. I need acknowledgement of the things I cannot do, and assistance that takes my personal circumstances into account in sorting out ongoing plans for managing this chronic condition. However, whenever I have tried to go through official channels, I have hit silence, enormous waiting times, and a sort of 'eh' attitude. Here is a PDF – I have just spent ten minutes trying to explain that brain fog means I cannot reliably understand communications anymore, including written ones, and that at its worst I stopped being able to read properly. Here are some painkillers – I have spent 10 minutes explaining that ibuprofen is no longer affecting the chest pain I have. I am told I can come back if the chest pain gets worse to discuss other pain management options. I am worried I will forget to do this or remember that I should but not have enough energy to fight with the e-consult form. Here is a set of breathing physio exercises to help with the breathlessness and the chest pain – this works when I am able to do them; however, due to pre-existing conditions, I have two other daily sets of physio I am supposed to complete, and I have a very limited amount of energy. I am in an endless loop of catch 22s that almost certainly has an exit that I could see if I was healthy. I am not healthy.

It does not feel as though there is anything I can do, so I remain at home. I take a lot of naps. I try to remember to top up my electricity meter key. I schedule a time to ring up the Department for Work and Pensions and ask about PIP. I prepare for the Post-Covid Unit appointment, although I don't know what it will be like at all or if they will be able to do anything other than give me the same advice I have had from my GP. I call friends and ask if they can do my laundry for me. It's relentless, and I am furious, and I do not want to talk about fucking lessons learned. I do not want to be an inspirational fucking story about overcoming blah blah blah blah blah. I don't want to meditate, or think positively, or look on the bright side. I want a coherent, cohesive, competent welfare system that doesn't take six months to get back to me. I want a health system that's properly funded and interlocked with the social welfare system and that ensures my GP has enough time to actually take care of me. I want a pay rise for all health workers and no privatisation of the NHS. I want consequences for the government that fucked this up. And, while I'm on a roll, I want universal basic income, and I want the vaccination patents to be waived, and I want the global minority to stop hoarding all the fucking Covid vaccinations and then turning around and acting surprised when we're hit with new variants.

I may never again find words as easily as I used to. I may spend the rest of my life walking into rooms and wondering what I am doing there, or forgetting conversations that I'm in the middle of and needing things repeated. I may never be able to walk more than three miles in one go again, or breathe properly, or go out in the cold. No one knows what recovery from long Covid looks like at this point. It would be a lot less stressful if it felt like anyone in charge was valuing human lives and wellbeing over money. I hate that I live in a world where a Flash Player video game had a better response to a global pandemic than actual world leaders.

Changing my relationship with my body
Sophie Hunter

March 2020. Just before the first lockdown, I started to feel odd – tight-chested, a bit dizzy and very tired. Nothing else. Because I'd just moved into our new house, which was a building site and full of brick dust, I assumed it was that and stress and nothing to worry about. First week of lockdown was juggling full-time work (suddenly all online) while coaxing two teens into home schooling and managing the builder, who was still working outside at a distance. Each Zoom call took more and more out of me and required more recovery. I worked like that for two weeks, feeling worse and worse, but thinking that if I *was* going to get Covid-19, I'd better get all my work in order first, so I could hand it on to a colleague! After two weeks, I realised I really couldn't go on, and was signed off sick for a fortnight (which was extended). It was such a relief to go to bed!

April 2020. My symptoms worsened after a week of being in bed – my breathing was worse and I began to get alarmed that I wasn't getting better. A friend had lent me a pulse-oximeter, which showed my oxygen levels were okay (which was brilliantly reassuring) but then the GP suggested I should go to A&E. That was a weird experience – being triaged in the car park because they didn't know whether to put me into the Covid side of the hospital or not. In the end, as I had no temperature or cough, I ended up in the non-Covid side, for a five-hour stay. They took chest x-rays and bloods and ECG and all sorts of other things, and finally decided that I must have had the virus, and this was the post-viral phase. They didn't test me for Covid-19 as 'it would only have been 60% effective', given I was past the infectious phase. There were lots of others in A&E that day who had similar symptoms, so the doctor felt he was beginning to see a pattern to the virus, and that recovery was taking a long time. Long Covid wasn't even named then.

June 2020. I go back to work. I'm slow. I still need to nap. Thank goodness for working at home and on Zoom. My symptoms continued unabated through the summer, and in October I decided that I needed to go away and be by myself. I went to a cottage in the Lake District and spent the week sleeping, walking, dreaming and painting. And I barely talked. I read the notebook that I had written in during the days in April when I was in bed and couldn't speak. There was *so much* in there! So many ideas of things I could do to support myself. When I got home from the Lakes, I decided to implement them all into my daily life… herbal remedies, rest, boundary setting, immersion in nature, being creative, stopping, making time for myself, listening to my body for the first time in my life. I found gentle Tai Chi exercises very helpful. It was slow; recovery happened step by step, and it took another 10 months before I really feel better. But along the way, I learnt so much about my relationship with my own health and wellbeing. It's been a journey!

My family
Sarah O'Connell

I have two children aged 11 and 7 with long Covid. My daughter was starting to show good signs of recovering from the ME she already had and was attending school part-time when she caught Covid and then long Covid. My son has never had any serious ill health issues but then he got Covid in August 2021, apparently mildly, and got it again in December and had a post-viral inflammatory response around Christmas. After that he became extremely unwell. I work with the campaign group Long Covid Kids,[5] and we are seeing a clear pattern of multiple cases of long Covid in some families, which suggests there may some role played by a genetic predisposition, as well as others where only one child in the family has it. I also have ME and am now dealing with long Covid too. (My mother also has ME and both of my sisters have had long Covid – one has recovered.) I was

---

5. For details of the groups mentioned here, see Resources at the end of the chapter.

prepared for some of the challenges of dealing with post-viral illness but when my son developed Paediatric Acute-onset Neuropsychiatric Syndrome (PANS), my world went upside down. On top of symptoms of extreme fatigue and pain, he's developed huge emotional and behavioural unpredictability and flares of temper and aggression, when, for example, he will scratch and kick and has even punched his sister in the face, causing her to bleed. The challenge of remaining calm and patient, of giving both children what they need, is taking its toll on my own health now.

I knew that we might struggle to get recognition from doctors (long Covid, and PANS in particular, are not well understood by many medical professionals), and so it proved, despite my being able to present a strong case for the PANS diagnosis. It was thanks to the PANS website that I found the only two doctors in Ireland qualified to help with this. To get help at a consultant level, we were advised to come to England. The whole trip cost us €3,000. I cannot work and my partner is feeling the huge burden of trying to keep our family afloat financially with these additional health needs.

The worst thing is not being understood. Family and friends don't ask questions or offer much support. I often think, if our children had any other serious illness, there would be more sympathy and support. Even the school, having been very good about my daughter, was more resistant when I said my son needed to attend part-time. Now he doesn't really even go out of the house much and has about an hour of good energy a day. It is impossible to go out for a family meal. Life is utterly unpredictable. I wake up thinking, will this be a good day or a bad day? I go to bed thinking tomorrow cannot be worse than today. And it often is!

What has kept me sane is my colleagues at Long Covid Kids, particularly one of the other reps whose daughter has PANS too. The PANS Facebook support group and charity have been amazing and I get a lot of support via Twitter. It feels sad that it is like this, but it is. I am never sure how much to tell other parents. I don't want them thinking we are weird or hypochondriacs.

My advice to other parents is to trust your instincts. You know your child. The doctors don't know everything. If you feel something is wrong, then don't let it drop. And reach out. The groups out there are full of people who really do understand what you are going through.

This has changed my life

I want to be able to share my experiences and contribute to the growing knowledge about long Covid. It has changed my life, and there are thousands of us.

I am 15 years old. Next year is my GCSE year and being ill could affect my whole future. I have always loved sport. Now I going to have to ask for some mitigation to be made for my PE practical, and other areas too. Sport is how I exercise, feel good about myself and socialise. That has all been taken away.

I got Covid at the beginning of September 2021 and it was pretty bad. I was the only one in my family to get it. I literally could not get off the sofa. I didn't want to eat. Food tasted weird as I had no sense of taste or smell, and I had a headache the whole time. Not just a headache, a monster headache. And I just couldn't think.

Then, in the two months that followed, most of those symptoms stayed, and I felt really anxious. I was worried about the future. Would I get better? Would I be able to do my exams? If not, how would that affect my whole life? Getting the vaccine was also very scary as some of the original symptoms reappeared and I thought I was going to get really ill all over again.

Getting close to Christmas, we began looking for more help. I was so, so tired all the time. I had brain fog and muscle and joint pain. We spoke to the GP. We have now seen quite a lot of doctors and they don't seem to understand. They tell me to pace myself. I try, but when you are struggling to even take a shower or clean your teeth and that doesn't seem to change, it is hard to know how to do this. Then you feel rubbish because you can't even look after yourself.

In the New Year we realised that I obviously had long Covid and that was tough. No one understands it fully. It is very hard to be taken seriously and get any real help. They just tell you it will get better, but they don't really know, and it is difficult to trust the advice you get. I was in grief when I realised I had it. It was so difficult to accept in so many ways.

We got my timetable reduced because I would just go into school, struggle through, half the time not really taking in what I was supposed to be learning, and then go home and sleep. No time to do any homework or things I enjoyed. Working shorter weeks has definitely helped with the energy levels and I am now worried about missing so many lessons. Some staff have been very understanding, like the person who rescheduled my timetable, but a lot of others don't really appreciate that this is not just about being a bit tired. I have not felt very supported or understood. Luckily my mum has been amazing. She will always listen to me. We have worked out for ourselves a few things that do seem to help, like supplements.

Friends don't really understand. They try. They ask me out for birthday meals or picnics and I just don't enjoy eating anymore. I hate the texture of a lot of food. In fact, eating has become a bit of an issue. Friends make a plan to do something with me and then I have to cancel because, when the time comes, I just feel too tired. This makes me feel very isolated.

No one seems able to help

My daughter was a healthy, very active nine-year-old – swimmer, kayaker and competitive trampolinist. She got Covid in February 2022. She now uses a wheelchair or bumshuffles on the floor, due to feeling dizzy and erratic heart rate, struggles to hold her head up because of headaches, cannot look at screens and is unable to attend school. Some nights she does not sleep at all. We have videoed her at night so we know this is true, despite trying herbal remedies, meditation tracks and other good sleep hygiene techniques. She is deathly pale, her lips are cracked. We have seen a number of doctors – most did not fully examine her. It took months to see a paediatrician. Some recommended trying to wake her up to establish a normal sleep routine. This made her worse. No one seems able to help us. Now they say she has post-viral fatigue. Long Covid Kids has been a life-saver but the doctors don't take any notice of all the information and experience being shared on that forum.

We live in Wales. This has turned out to be an issue as the Welsh health service has a policy of surgery phlebotomists not taking blood from minors. This has made getting tests much more difficult for her.

I am a fighter. I keep making phone calls, pushing for things to be done, trying to get different specialists to talk to one another. Today when I rang up the doctor, they agreed to arrange another blood test. Then they asked me what I wanted it to be for! I don't have a degree in medicine. You feel on your own. It's taking its toll. I am tired. I have two other children. This will be a very, very long road for our family.

What about the other parents who don't have the confidence to push? The ones who feel intimidated when they talk to a doctor. What about those children?

Even the honk of a car horn puts me in agony

Samir T

I am 12 years old and I caught Covid in September 2021 just after I started my new school. For a couple of months, I had random ailments and high fevers, and then, around February, my symptoms settled into a pattern.

Unimaginable pain was caused by any vibrations or walking; even burping or yawning set me off. I had dizziness, headaches, burning hands and feet and could not control my body temperature. I got muscle spasms often; I couldn't even sit in a chair without them starting. The pain of these would be enough to make me scream.

After trips to GPs and other doctors, I finally got referred to the long Covid clinic and went for observation. I have been taking antihistamines, vitamin D, iron, multivitamins, probiotics and melatonin at night.

I tried going into school for just a few lessons at a time, but it was too much. Computing used to be my favourite subject. It took me an hour to get there, and I just cannot manage it. We are worried about how I will manage school in the future. I have barely been able to talk to my friends. Once the doctors told the school about long Covid, they allowed me to attend lessons online, but later I was given a tutor for shorter lessons as I could not focus for long. The hospital is a long way away too.

I loved swimming and bike rides before, and when we went on holiday to Cornwall I would try to climb the cliffs as high as I could. Now I dread going out of the house. It is too painful and unpredictable. I spend most of the day on the sofa because ordinary chairs set me off. If I have to travel in a car, it puts me in agony from the vibrations, from the car's engine to the bumps on the road to the honk of a horn.

Now I read a lot. I have recently been reading about mythologies. I especially like Rick Riordan's books,[6] the *Percy Jackson & the Olympians*

---

6. All those listed here are published by Penguin Books in the UK.

series (2005–09) and the pentalogies *The Heroes of Olympus* (2010–14) and *The Trials of Apollo* (2016–20).

My mum joined Long Covid Kids and has found it very helpful. I have just got accepted now, so I will be able to join the private chat. I play games every week with people on there and it is good to be with people my age who understand.

What's wrong with me?

I am 14, and this is my story of how I got diagnosed with long Covid.

One morning, I woke up in pain and could not move my body. Ever since, I have been in pain most days, leaving me unable to walk and function normally. We had to call an ambulance a couple of times because I just could not get out of bed and I couldn't move. I felt so frightened.

At first some doctors said I had viral arthritis, as I had a virus a month before it all started. The hardest thing for me has been months of not knowing why I feel like this, which only changed when I got referred to a long Covid clinic. They eliminate all the things it might be and, when they had done all their tests, they told me that I had long Covid, which was a surprise as officially I have never tested positive for Covid.

I like skating, going for walks and going out to meet my friends, and I also had a job in a café in the park. I have had to give up these activities and I'm not seeing my friends nearly as much as I want to.

I now have to pace myself. I need to reduce stress, otherwise my muscles seize up and brain fog sets in. Things that used to take time now take much longer and I now need to accept that.

Morning routines are taking prescribed vitamins and painkillers, and then I take my time with moving and getting up. Most mornings consist of needing a helping hand – if I stumble, I need to grab walls to steady myself, which is why my dad has given up work to look after me. He now helps me get to school and drives me in, as the walk is too far to even attempt.

My school has been very helpful as my classroom used to be up three flights of stairs, so they have moved me to the ground floor. I am lucky that they have a specially built complex for children with mobility and learning challenges. I am so grateful for their support and understanding – they allow me to get to school in my own time, and I do try to attend any lessons I am able to walk to in other parts of the school, to be with my friends.

If I go for a walk, my mum and dad bring a wheelchair we have got and, when I know I have done enough, I ride back in it.

The best advice I have been given, and have also figured out for myself, is to pace yourself, take your time and work to no more than 80% of your old self, or you will suffer the next day. When you are able to take your time, with no pressure to rush, your anxiety levels drop and you can do more!

It is good knowing that, and that I am not alone. My family has joined a few groups on social media to share experiences and to help each other. It's tiring living like this, but it is getting better day by day. I just wish the old me would hurry up and come back.

Commentary
Lesley Macniven

I'm a founding member of Long Covid Support (LCS),[7] a charity formed by people with long Covid. It began as a Facebook group in May 2020 and by April 2022 was nudging 52,000 users across the globe. It is fitting that the story of the family of the founder of the Facebook group, Claire Hastie, begins this chapter.

The stories here reveal the all-consuming impact of long Covid on people's lives and on families – the having to cope alone, isolated from friends and family, and being cared for by your own children. I felt lucky to have a partner at home. I don't think I'd have made it if I'd had to rely on my two girls. I (half) jest – however, having to confront your own mortality and desperately try to put your affairs in order while feeling so ill is a common theme we hear in people's accounts.

On 13 March 2020, Dominic Cummings, then advisor to the Prime Minister, wrote the chilling phrase 'Who do we not save?' on a whiteboard in a Downing Street meeting,[8] 10 days before the first lockdown.

7. For details of the groups mentioned here, see Resources at the end of the chapter.
8. www.bbc.co.uk/news/health-57254654

According to the October 2022 ONS Long Covid monthly update,[9] 2.3 million (3.5% of the UK population) had long Covid at the beginning of the previous month. For some 72%, their day-to-day life is 'adversely affected' by the condition; 15% say they are limited 'a lot'. The data also reveal that 74,000 of those people living with long Covid today, including me, many of those I work with at LCS and most of those whose stories are told here, became infected during those final few weeks leading up to the first lockdown.

The decisions taken by Downing Street in this period – and its indecisions – were critical to the government's failure to stop the spread of the first wave of Covid to the many thousands who are now caught in its tail – those with long Covid. It was the projected 4,000 Covid deaths a day, precipitating a collapse of the NHS, that prompted Cummings' scrawl, 'Who do we not save?', and the *Stay Home and Save the NHS* public message.

But was the likelihood of ongoing chronic illness, of long Covid, ever anticipated? The single decision-making criterion seemed to be 'death or survival'. Who could be saved? And now we are in the midst of a second pandemic – of people who have been ill with Covid and are not recovering within the projected 12 weeks. It was those who were afflicted with long Covid who named this phenomenon[10] and drew it to the attention of the world.

I contracted Covid-19 on 10 March 2020, pre-lockdown. Before the pandemic, I was an organisational development professional, instigating and supporting change at organisation, team and individual levels, with a specific interest in diversity and inclusion. It was inevitable that, witnessing how existing inequalities were being exacerbated by the pandemic and the emergence of a whole new, invisibilised and marginalised group, I would become a 'couch-based activist' for my own and others' cause.

No fewer than 62 different symptoms have been associated with long Covid, ranging from the most common – breathlessness, fatigue, brain fog, insomnia, chest pain, loss of sense of smell and taste,

---

9. www.ons.gov.uk/peoplepopulationandcommunity/healthandsocialcare/conditions anddiseases/bulletins/prevalenceofongoingsymptomsfollowingcoronaviruscovid19 infectionintheuk/6october2022

10. https://twitter.com/elisaperego78/status/1395443525437829120?s=20&t=Yietup_ RzeDSBrKx0omGMA

muscle pain – through to loss of hair, loss of libido, and psychological sequellae, such as anxiety, flattened mood, anorexia and depression. Many, of course, have more than one symptom. And the prevalence of long Covid seems to be growing with each wave. One in 10 are too unwell to work (Subramanian et al, 2022).

Research has separated those with the varied symptoms into three 'classes': 80.0% have a spectrum of symptoms including pain, fatigue and rash; 5.8% report longstanding cough, shortness of breath and phlegm, and 14.2% report depression, anxiety, insomnia and brain fog. But across all three groups, women and people living in poverty are still the most likely to be affected (Subramanian et al., 2022).

Minimal data collection and testing in the early days no doubt contributed to patients' common experience of feeling patronised and, worse, rampant medical gaslighting. Sketchy data allowed the medical profession and policy makers to downplay and dismiss individual testimony. Describing symptoms dismissively as 'self-reported' allows an assumption of psychological, not physiological, causes and justifies inaction. It was ever thus with 'disorders' that medicine cannot explain. People with chronic fatigue syndrome/ME are only too painfully aware of this. Our hope is that their experience may inform how the health service goes forward with long Covid. Or will we too be ignored and our knowledge and experience dismissed as unreliable and untested?

Being repeatedly told to ignore our own instincts, our reality, is deeply traumatic. So too is having your sanity questioned and doubted. How do you sleep when you know that, when symptoms feel anything but 'mild', you may not actually wake up next day? I marvel at the resilience of those who have survived and are still here today, telling their stories – largely because they found groups, discovered they were not alone and gained the courage to do so.

Embryonic online connections calcified into the backbone of a movement to influence the deluded decision-makers who led us into this global tragedy and catch the thousands who were falling between the cracks in healthcare provision. Without each other, I'm certain we would have lost many more. Searching for interim solutions, rehab, research and recognition for each other helped us endure and gave us a sense of purpose. We naïvely thought that, if we spoke out, help would reach us once the death rates started to fall. Meantime, in lieu of medical care and while research groups applied for grants, we facilitated peer first aid.

We tried to warn the public, as the chronic illness and ME community had warned us, to rest and be wary of exercise-based advice.

We also had input to the NICE clinical guideline that, notably, states you can be given a clinical diagnosis of long Covid by a GP based on your symptoms and no Covid antibody test is required (NICE, 2022).

Research

Bio-medical research is revealing multiple impacts of long Covid, including organ damage, neurological effects and microclots persisting in the blood of those who have been ill the longest (see, for example, Proal & VanElzakker, 2021).

Clinicians anticipate that many different bodily systems may be affected, sometimes simultaneously, meaning widely available effective medical treatment is likely to be some way off. And in the absence of treatments that do work, treatments that don't are being marketed to the vulnerable and desperate. People are travelling abroad to have unproven treatments such as 'blood washing'. And where are the trials of promising long Covid treatments? There are vanishingly few, when surely, given the scale of the problem, this should be a worldwide, co-ordinated endeavour?

Filling the vacuum of data on the growing long Covid pandemic, patient groups have provided each other with support and, increasingly, provided the medical community with data. We need them now to take it from here by instigating the necessary research. But we don't just need research into the biological causes, in search of the elusive drug that will effect the miracle cure. As long as they fail to find the cause, the plight and testimonies of those with long Covid will continue to be dismissed, disbelieved and ignored. We need our testimonies of what we find works to help us live with long Covid to be researched so that these valuable insights can be evidenced and shared.

Analysis of long Covid groups' patient-led research is publicly available, and there are dedicated patient involvement groups to help researchers and funding organisations consider research questions and funding decisions. Patient and public involvement in research to find treatments has increased, but there is frustration among survivors that such research remains very much in its infancy. Instead patients have become 'experts by experience', while clinicians and researchers catch up with what we have learned. It's time to speed up this painfully slow process to get meaningful answers and treatment.

And the numbers of people with long Covid are still growing. At great cost to individuals, families and communities, and also to the national economy. In addition to 74,000 of us who developed long Covid in the first wave, another 784,000 joined us in the second wave. More recently, the total has grown to 2.3 million (October, 2022).[11] And still the numbers grow, as the virus continues to mutate and spread.

Rehabilitation

I am Chair of the LCS Employment Group. Working with the TUC, we gathered evidence from people with long Covid on wider employment and welfare issues, revealing the widespread lack of understanding of the condition and bias and stigma in workplaces (TUC, 2021).

We need more inclusive general working practices and reasonable adjustments in the workplace. The relapsing and remitting nature and cognitive impacts of long Covid affect workers' stamina and high-level thinking, so may require specialised risk assessments. Our finding is that integrated multidisciplinary solutions are needed to help people return to the workplace safely and with a better chance of staying well.

How many have fallen into poverty as a result of being disabled by long Covid and are being abandoned to languish? How many already living in poverty are being driven further into destitution?

Frontline workers, our 'pandemic heroes', now struck down by long Covid, should not be regarded as unavoidable, unfortunate collateral damage. This jarring example shows how devastatingly let down so many who are left with the long-lasting impact of Covid now feel. Add in the current hike in the cost of living and disappearance of the 'We're all in it together' community spirit. Is there still time to pause, re-evaluate and refocus on what's most important? Attention to health, wellbeing and how we support those in need could be a key measure of the UK's progress.

11.www.ons.gov.uk/peoplepopulationandcommunity/healthandsocialcare/ conditionsanddiseases/bulletins/prevalenceofongoingsymptomsfollowingcoronavirus covid19infectionintheuk/6october2022

Living with Covid, we are all playing the Russian roulette of Covid-19 infection. More and more of us are falling prey to the virus, yet it has not galvanised change in how our benefits, employment support and medical services respond. If we join forces across every sector, occupation and demographic, we can argue to do things differently, a better future could come out of a horrific time, there'd be a greater focus on quality of life, and patient campaign groups could simply become friendship groups.

No one should be left behind.

References

NICE. (2022). *Covid-19 rapid guideline: Managing the long-term effects of COVID-19*. NICE. www.nice.org.uk/guidance/ng188/resources/covid19-rapid-guideline-managing-the-longterm-effects-of-covid19-pdf-51035515742

Proal, A.D. & VanElzakker, M.B. (2021). Long COVID or post-acute sequelae of COVID-19 (PASC): An overview of biological factors that may contribute to persistent symptoms. *Frontiers in Microbiology, 12.* doi.org/10.3389/fmicb.2021.698169

Subramanian, A., Nirantharakumar, K., Hughes, S. et al (2022). Symptoms and risk factors for long COVID in non-hospitalized adults. *Nature Medicine, 28,*1706–1714.

TUC. (2021). *Workers' experience of long Covid: A TUC report.* TUC. www.tuc.org.uk/sites/default/files/2021-06/Formatted%20version%20of%20Long%20Covid%20report%20-%20v1.3.pdf

---

Pre-Covid, Lesley Macniven was a freelance consultant, passionate about workplace equality, working with clients to deliver diversity, inclusion and change projects. Lesley is a founding member of the patient-led support and campaign group, Long Covid Support. During 2021, Lesley worked with the Society of Occupational Medicine, the TUC and her professional body, the CIPD, in her role as Chair of the Long Covid Support Employment Group, and as a consultant with occupational professional colleagues at www.longcovidwork.co.uk. Lesley also runs creative writing 'workshops for wellbeing' and literary events where the voices of people with long Covid and the narrative around this 'second pandemic' can be heard.

Commentary
Kodama Allende, TeachersWithCovidUK

I am a secondary school teacher, one of those thousands of frontline workers who not only got Covid but is now suffering with long Covid and having to fight battles on what seems like every front to stay financially afloat, recover my health and return to work.

I caught Covid in the autumn of 2020, before there was routine testing. So, when my symptoms persisted long after I was supposed to have recovered, the reaction from my school and colleagues was often one of disbelief, resentment and even spite. And, as I know from other teachers' stories, I am not alone.

I was struggling to breathe, my body had been fighting for oxygen for months and was getting weaker, nothing was functioning properly, and especially not my brain. I had tried to return to work but was clearly not well enough – I could barely walk or breathe or speak above a whisper.

Everyone in the school was under a huge amount of pressure trying to put in place the constantly changing rules and regulations imposed by the government. We were all struggling with the impact of pandemic. As I was the only specialist teacher in my A level subjects, my being off sick was adding even more stress to my colleagues. I started getting formal letters from school, questioning whether I had even had Covid and clearly not understanding the severity of my symptoms. I can understand this, to an extent. Sympathy turned to resentment, adding immensely to my confusion, isolation and overwhelming sense of losing myself physically and emotionally.

I needed help but my union, like everyone else, didn't understand the nature of long Covid and what I needed. I was in no fit state to fight what had become a battle with my employer. Even the medical community had still to understand what was happening to people with these long-term symptoms, never mind why or how to fix them. The lack of medical evidence meant it was impossible to get concessions, adjustments and help. Thousands like me were left being swirled around in a bureaucracy that didn't have any forms, procedures or protocols that fitted our circumstances. I was left clinging onto not only my precious, inefficient breaths, but also to my income, as the sole earner for a family of three, and my home and my will to live.

Eventually I realised this couldn't go on and I started looking for help. I searched the internet and social media and couldn't find what I was looking for, so I decided to start a Facebook group, TeachersWithCovidUK.[12] As our numbers grew steadily, we became aware we were far from alone and began to help each other navigate this journey. We were all experiencing similar issues and became familiar with employment law, disability rights and much more. I discovered I was relatively lucky: some people's experiences were truly shocking. For example, one teacher asked to have classes downstairs as they were too weak to climb the two flights to their usual classroom. They were refused, even though this is standard practice if a pupil has broken a leg. In the end, their employment was terminated on grounds of ill health, instead of making reasonable adjustments so this experienced teacher with management responsibilities could continue in their role. This was almost certainly illegal, but when you are fighting a chronic illness, you simply don't have the ability to stand up for yourself.

When the majority of teachers were (and are) catching Covid at work, this poor treatment by employers and inadequate support from the unions seems particularly cruel. I watched people going downhill, losing their job, partner and home, and being left in poverty with no quality of life or hope. Yet a few teachers in the group reported amazing colleagues and employers. They were allowed very gentle phased returns, provided with mobility aids, found flowers on their desks in the mornings, and were treated humanely. Every single one of these teachers gradually got better and is still teaching. It is amazing how much difference a little kindness and accommodation can make – and it makes so much more sense economically.

Sharing our experiences in the Facebook group has enabled us to see emerging patterns of symptoms and helpful treatments. This is a new disease, and no one really understands it fully, but as Lesley Macniven points out, too little research is being done that involves the people who are best placed to know these things – people with long Covid. We will only begin to understand by gathering data and carrying out more research. In the meantime, preventing people getting Covid

12. www.facebook.com/groups/TeacherswithCovidUK/about

in the first place remains crucial. It was a long time before pupils were required to wear masks. It was always blatantly obvious that schools would be hot-beds of transmission. But government advice was incredibly slow to shift from mitigation measures to prevent the spread of droplets to steps to prevent airborne transmission, and even these have now been abandoned. Ventilation is not being put in place and there remains resistance to this. The majority of UK classrooms remain poorly ventilated and overcrowded, particularly in deprived areas. People working in the education sector are 37% more likely to get Covid than any other workers.

We are now in the midst of an epidemic of long Covid – at the time of writing, some 2.3 million people in the UK have long Covid, 514,000, of whom have had it for at least two years.[13]

And it is small wonder that teachers and other education-sector staff are in the top three professions with the highest number of long Covid sufferers, along with health and social care and medical staff. In March 2022, the ONS estimated that 3.79 per cent of the UK teaching and education and social care sectors were living with self-reported long Covid of any duration, higher than people in the healthcare sector (3.69 per cent). Rates were also rising faster than in any other sector, 'likely reflecting increased exposure to Covid-19 in these sectors'.[14]

Of course, it is not only the staff that are affected by Covid. Even though children are significantly less likely to die from Covid, they are getting long Covid, as the stories included here tell us. School absence rates are now at record levels. In July 2022, 25% of all students in England's state primary and secondary schools were absent (for any reason) and levels of student absence across the academic year are significantly higher than pre-pandemic levels.[15]

With regard specifically to long Covid, in the academic year 2021–2022, around a fifth of Year 13 students in day schools in the

---

13. www.ons.gov.uk/peoplepopulationandcommunity/healthandsocialcare/
conditionsanddiseases/bulletins/prevalenceofongoingsymptomsfollowingcoronavirus
covid19infectionintheuk/6october2022

14. www.ons.gov.uk/peoplepopulationandcommunity/healthandsocialcare/
conditionsanddiseases/datasets/alldatarelatingtoprevalenceofongoingsymptoms
followingcoronaviruscovid19infectionintheuk/3march2022

15. https://explore-education-statistics.service.gov.uk/find-statistics/attendance-in-
education-and-early-years-settings-during-the-coronavirus-covid-19-outbreak

UK had missed more than four weeks of their crucial final A-level year for this reason. In May 2022, some 100,000 children aged 2–16 had long Covid, 22,000 of whom had symptoms that had lasted more than a year.[16]

Parents are watching their children endure distressing symptoms. Online support forums are full of harrowing stories and desperate pleas for help from parents who are beside themselves when there are so few answers from the medical profession. Parents are having to give up work to care for their sick children and are trying desperately to find the answers they are not getting from overstretched medical staff.

Very little is being done to implement mitigations we know work – clean air being one that would improve every pupil's learning and alertness, as well as halt the spread of all airborne diseases. It is pure negligence not to install the relatively cheap, scientifically proven-effective HEPA air-cleaning filters (or equivalent systems) in all classrooms, at the very least.

Covid is devastating. Long Covid is devastating and goes on much, much longer, with huge implications for these children's future lives. We have the knowledge and the means to prevent this suffering. So why are successive governments choosing not to?

Kodama Allende lives and works in the south east of England. Kodama Allende is a pen name to protect her identity. She is a film-maker, photographer, animator and educator, with more than 20 years' experience. She now teaches curriculum subjects in state schools and privately, and trains adults in the practical aspects of film-making. Her son became very ill age 13 and Kodama worked tirelessly to correctly diagnose and treat him when the NHS had given up on him. His initial diagnoses was ME but Kodama eventually diagnosed Lyme disease, which has now been successfully treated by a specialist in America. On discovering the history, politics and mistreatment of ME patients, she actively joined the many charities and support groups campaigning for improvements in education, understanding and medical treatments to

---

16. www.ons.gov.uk/peoplepopulationandcommunity/healthandsocialcare/conditions anddiseases/datasets/alldatarelatingtoprevalenceofongoingsymptomsfollowingcorona viruscovid19infectionintheuk

serve these patients better. She is now co-chair of a support group for people with ME. She caught Covid while teaching in March 2020, and still experiences debilitating symptoms, but has used her experience to help fast track a beneficial approach to long Covid.

Resources

Long Covid patient-led support groups

Long Covid Kids. *www.longcovidkids.org*

Long Covid Physio. Useful resources on pacing and other forms of rehab. *https://longcovid.physio*

Long Covid Support (private group). *www.facebook.com/groups/longcovid*

Long Covid Support (public page). *www.longcovid.org*

Long Covid Support Employment Group. *https://longcovidwork.co.uk/2021/ 12/07/vra-2021-special-recognition-award-and-the-launch-of-long-covid-work*

Long Covid Scotland. *www.longcovid.scot*

Long Covid Wales. *https://twitter.com/LongCovidWales?s=20&t=obstWWcj 4rwiSopDpQ2jWA*

Long Covid Work. Source of information on returning to work and welfare. *https://longcovidwork.co.uk*

PANS/PANDAS Parent Support. Support group for parents of children with PANS and PANDAS. *www.facebook.com/groups/PANDASParentsGroup*

PANS PANDAS UK. Support and campaign group. *www.panspandasuk.org*

Teachers with Covid UK. *www.facebook.com/groups/TeacherswithCovidUK/ about*

Yoga and Meditation for Gentle Covid Recovery. Facebook group. *www. facebook.com/groups/1095053437543132*

Video

Paisley Book Festival. Stories that kept us sane: A long Covid writer's showcase. *www.youtube.com/watch?v=zoq0COYA4cQ*

Apps

InsightTimer. Free app for sleep, anxiety and stress with hundreds of guided meditations. *https://insighttimer.com/en-gb*

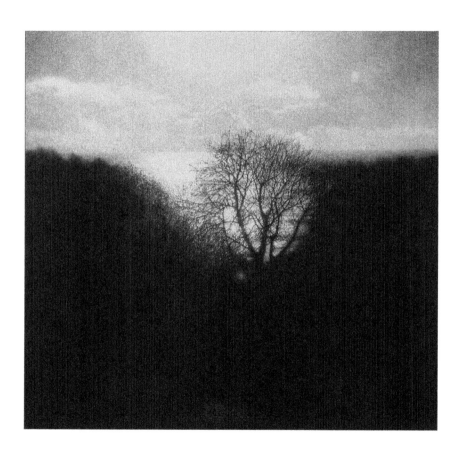

6.

Emerging

Covid-19 diary

Diane Harris

These words come from the diary I kept all through lockdown.

'My name is Diane Harris and I am 80 years of age. I never got my party for my birthday, but I am alive.

'Isolation – how to cope with it? Take one day at a time. Easy to say, hard to do. Three months inside, no mixing with friends and family. Not true. Today's technology means you are only ever a phone call away. The biggest thing is staying positive.

'My daughter has come up with an idea, so I painted a rainbow and sellotaped it to my outside window. I live in a flat which is sheltered housing. So now people will either think I have flipped or be astounded at my talent. Opposite me is a nursing home. Maybe my rainbow will bring a smile to someone's face.'

Community stories

400 unsung heroes

Sarah Anthony

Covid was coming. It was just at that point when it was very bad in Italy and clearly coming our way. I have extended family in Italy, so I knew what was happening wasn't just media hype.

I am a project manager, and I was on maternity leave. I had a little girl who had just turned three, and a 10-month-old baby. At the weekends, my husband and I would take it in turns to go away after lunch to have a coffee and read a book for an hour and get some peace. This particular time, I was reading the news. I knew this was coming to Abingdon. I'm a practising Christian and I was thinking, 'What can I do? I can't help those in hospitals. I'm not a medic, but people, particularly older people, could be stuck at home in a lockdown without being able to get supplies or help.' I thought, 'There must be other people in the town thinking this.' So I put a post on the town Facebook saying I was worried and wondering if we could do something, asking if anyone else felt the same.

Within minutes I had 10 or 12 responses, so I set up a Facebook group and invited people to spread the word. By the end of the hour, 100 people were signed up. Then I had to sheepishly go home and tell my husband what I had started! By the evening, there were about 1,000 volunteers and next morning a designer was creating postcards for taking door to door, signposting help, and a printer had volunteered to print 17,000 of them for free. It all moved so fast at the start and so did the Covid. We set up a face-to-face meeting for the Thursday – it seems crazy to think we did that now! Then we realised this was clearly a terrible idea and we'd need to do it all virtually. But it is tricky when you are working with total strangers. People started offering to do all sorts of things. Luckily for me, some people also volunteered to help with the organising! So we divided Abingdon up and volunteers put postcards through every single door giving details of a street contact who could respond to requests or pass it on to another volunteer in their neighbourhood.

There were lots of disasters along the way and it was crazy but great. We learned fast!

In the first 12-week lockdown we had more than 400 volunteers and carried out more than 4,000 individual responses. Those responses could be anything from queuing three hours for one person's shopping or driving someone to hospital. We worked out that people had collectively volunteered hours totalling nearly one entire working year! We negotiated access arrangements with supermarkets and got jackets printed so supermarkets and residents knew who we were. The Co-op wanted to offer deliveries, but they were not set up to do this, so they asked us to create a team of volunteer drivers. So did the food bank. Then the council got in touch because they did not have the capacity to carry out the plans proposed by central government. They asked for help, and we formed a local government council emergency response team. As time went on, we uncovered people facing really difficult circumstances, caused or exacerbated by Covid, and we were able to signpost them to other places too.

I guess it was a bit like what they say about the Blitz spirit during the war. People wanted to help. They would say, 'I feel really helpless but this is something I can do.' Some had been furloughed and suddenly had a lot of time and skills to share. They thought, 'I can be useful here.' It became a virtuous circle. WhatsApp groups got set up for streets and they had virtual street parties, and then had real ones when lockdown lifted.

I think all of us involved made new connections and friendships with people we didn't know before, and it's amazing to think that, if another disaster happened, the people of Abingdon would rally together again. Being involved made a terrible time that little bit better.

I met my neighbour
Julie Kay, Wirral Older People's Parliament

In the summer of 2020, I met my neighbour properly, as Covid meant we were suddenly saying hello and having little chats on the doorstep as she went to the local shop.

Being known
Sarah Grylls

I always knew I was extremely lucky to live in this row of 16 terraced cottages, which share a small green. The physical environment is lovely, and neighbourliness is the norm.

I had a few other resources and supports throughout the lockdowns, but even so, this neighbourliness, the people, the space and the messages, helped no end. I've learned some things about myself. First, that for me there is something calming and warming about knowing and being known in my community – not deeply, that would be terrifying, but lightly, cheerfully, consistently. This sense of belonging was there before the pandemic, and it was there even more strongly during it, when my need was greater.

Second, that I need to feel engaged with the world, to act and have an impact on it, in order to keep my sense of self intact. For many of us who are retired, the pandemic was simpler than for those having to make decisions or adaptations about travel, mixing with strangers, caring, studying, earning. We simply had to stay out of the way. I recognise my privilege, but I also found this dreary, depressing and confidence sapping. I did quite a lot of exercise and a little voluntary work, but still, if I'd not had our anytime access to green space and my neighbours to think about and communicate with, I would have felt even more hemmed in, squashed and unnecessary.

And finally, that it was important to me to hear and understand how others were making sense of what was happening, to talk about different lives, different hopes and priorities and different decisions. No amount of reading or viewing unknown people's versions of events in the media can compete with listening to neighbours talk about themselves, their families, their experiences and their opinions. I learned a lot, and definitely used other people's wisdom to help me plot my way through the two years.

A village response
Jude Bishop

Our small village in Devon has always been community minded and during lockdown it really rose to the occasion. A phone befriending scheme was set up in response to the first lockdown and more than 1,000 calls were made to those in isolation. The volunteers came in response to a village-wide callout for support. The South Brent and District Caring office co-ordinated the connections and, two years on, many of the volunteers have maintained their friendships with those they helped during the lockdown. With the easing of Covid restrictions, some of the recipients have started to attend lunch club and friendship groups.

We set up a food bank and a core team of five volunteers with complementary skills was put together to support those facing financial hardship. The two towns either side of us usually provided this support, but not being able to travel meant we had households facing a food shortage. We got local grants and donations of money and food from individuals and local shops. And we moved fast! From the first meeting to delivering our first food parcel took a mere three weeks, including getting a flyer to 1,000 households in the village and nearby hamlets. We operated for six months, from March to the end of August 2021, when restrictions were lifted and people could access their usual food bank. We distributed more than 63 parcels, which supported 183 people all told. It really is amazing what you can do when you pull together.

Food for mind and body
Dionne Gbasai

At Manchester Mind, we had to adapt our services and close the café, and instead we began distributing emergency meals cooked from vegetables grown on our allotment. The food we made to distribute became little lunches of hope, as simple as they were. I tried to pack each one with a little bit of dignity and put a smile inside. The kitchen became a hub of hope, filled with our brilliant staff team and amazing volunteers. All of us working to alleviate the stress and shame of people in the Manchester area experiencing food poverty. The pandemic has been a time of great uncertainty but also one of discovery. One service user said they had learned that there is no shame in asking for help and that there are many who need help and many more who needed help way before the pandemic. Volunteers with the food programme benefitted too. One wrote to us, 'Towards the end of the pandemic, I started to become very low, I didn't have a reason to get out of bed or do anything, so having the opportunity to go and help cook and prepare food with a lovely team really boosted my mood and gave me energy for the rest of the day.' And so, of course, did recipients of the food. One of them said to us, 'I don't know how to express my gratitude for your mental health support and help with the nice meals too. But most of all, I don't feel lonely. I have had more visitors in this week than in the last three months.'

Walk and talk
Linda

When my mum left to go to my sister's house to be looked after, I was on my own in the house for the first time. I was 40 then. Mum had dementia and I work full time, so that's what had to happen. Very sadly, 10 years later, she died of Covid in her care home. I was devastated.

I always say I am on my own but not lonely. I have a lot of good friends and a job I like. I am also a chronic asthmatic. So when Covid hit, I had to stay home. And then it was not so easy. I did not know what to do with myself. I had started a local friends group to get together, share information and so on, but now there were restrictions. We used to meet in the park, all women from all backgrounds, but then we couldn't. I tried WhatsApp and it was good, but I wanted to see people and get some exercise. I am lucky, I have a dog and a garden, but he is 18 and does not walk far now. So I suggested Walk and Talk, one to one. Meeting people and going for a walk. It was great. We saw new plants and birds, went to parks we had never visited, and talked. We all had different backgrounds and experiences – Bangladeshi, Afro-Caribbean, English, Muslim. We learn from each other. There's no judgement.

I know it helped me. I think my mental health would have been badly affected otherwise. It's just therapeutic, being together, walking and talking. One guy joined in who had just moved here from Italy. He got to meet people, which would have been really hard otherwise. Now we are all going to walk all the local parks in a day. Walk, cycle, go by wheelchair. There are 32 parks, and lots of them don't really get used much. One lady said she has got fitter, lost weight and walks faster. We keep each other going. When I am with someone, I am not just focusing on me. I go out twice a week. Sometimes we walk 15 miles. And I encourage people to take off their shoes and socks and walk on the grass. Have you tried it? It's great.

Online prayers

Rana Ibrahim, Iraqi Women Art and War (IWAW) group
I did a lot of things in lockdown. I got the chance to develop my own work as a collage artist. I had been doing art regularly with a group of women from Iraq here in the UK and we had a WhatsApp group. When lockdown came, it was hard to encourage the women to stay connected, but we found ways. I learned how to use Zoom and that really worked for us, and it meant we could be together with women artists in Iraq too. Some of them were women who had gone back from the UK. So we were connecting with our homeland and our family and friends there. We ran workshops during Refugee Week, and we talked about violence against women. It got a lot worse everywhere during lockdown. A lot of young girls were in danger. It is important to speak about these things.

And we cooked. All of us had to cook – every day. So I thought, 'Let's do something with this.' So we started filming ourselves cooking and talking about our recipes. I translated the recipes. It was very popular all over the world. We met new people this way. We wrote a poem together and read it out on local radio. And then Ramadan came and as we still could not come together as a community in our usual ways, I met with women and children everyday online to pray and say Duaa, and we made pictures of the many different names of Allah. There are a hundred and we did not complete them all. Inshallah we will next time. And I am sure I will go on using Zoom in my work to stay connected. **www.iwaw19.com**

Learning to offer support services online
Ruth Rosselson, resilience co-ordinator

I work for Manchester Mind, a mental health charity. My work is focused on delivering group interventions – different courses to help people build resilience and learn tools and techniques to help their mental health. One of the key elements to my resilience courses is the peer support. When everything shut down in March 2020, I was left feeling adrift. How could I continue to support people in this way when we couldn't even be in the same room together?

As I began to settle into working at home, I realised the importance of being able to offer something online. Something straightforward and simple for people to access – simple mindfulness meditations and calming techniques to help with the anxiety and stress nearly everyone was experiencing. These sessions were short, open to anyone and free. After a few weeks, we began to get a core of regulars, and I was pleased to find a sense of community building, and surprised that people were often very open, even to a bunch of strangers in rooms across the city.

I was pleased that I could still facilitate a safe, friendly and warm environment online. I helped some people use Zoom for the first time and made sure that people felt comfortable, despite feeling unsure of the technology. Using breakouts is a challenge – I'm used to overhearing conversations from the small groups and reading the room in terms of energy and body language to ensure that I address any issues for those who are struggling. I couldn't do that in the same way with the online courses, where breakouts were private. And I definitely didn't get to know people as well as I used to. Still, I did my best, checking in with people after a session if I sensed they were struggling, for example.

The best thing about Covid is that it forced me into exploring online delivery. A large number of people who attended would never have managed to get to an in-person course, even if it had been run locally to them. There was an extremely agoraphobic man who rarely left his home, for example; others with severe social anxiety felt brave enough to contribute, but not to have their cameras on, and there was a large number of people with chronic pain, fatigue or mobility issues that prevented them coming to an in-person course. Many of these people were isolated even before Covid. An 86-year-old woman who joined on her iPad fed back that her stress and anxiety had reduced and she was feeling less isolated because of the course. Another woman told me that it was the first support she'd received where she felt really understood. Some groups even continued to meet online after the course had finished.

I've just run my first in-person session, and it's highlighted what I've really missed these past two years – people getting to know each other before the session over coffee, for example, or walking home together afterwards. People are able to interject and reassure each other a lot more easily than if they had to unmute or put their hand up to do so on Zoom. I also already feel a sense of their personalities a lot quicker and more easily. It's clear that a hybrid form of delivery will be the way forward, ensuring that people have the choice of attending online or in person and that, whichever medium they choose, they will leave feeling supported, and connected to others and with some tools and techniques to help them along their way.

Friday frolics

Friday frolics began in lockdown when I took Mum her shopping. It started with a cup of tea in the garden on a Friday afternoon and developed into a glass of prosecco. My daughter, who had been learning to drive and was forced to stop, cottoned on to this, and so she would drive to Grandma's as a practice and I, of course, would always drive home… Prosecco and grandma's influence had everything to do with this! The weeks went by merrily on Friday afternoons with prosecco and jigsaws… so many jigsaws, the occasional dance and dog walk, and the tradition continues as my daughter still FaceTimes and frolics from university today. The experience brought three generations of women closer and Friday frolics will be a 'thing' in our family now forever.

All scrubbed up

Sophy Thomas

Early lockdown in 2020. I watched passively as hospitals were filling, NHS staff over-stretched. A social media post caught my eye about making scrubs for NHS staff, who were in desperate need. The project was started by Ashleigh Lindsell in Cambridgeshire. She was working as a nurse full time and sewing. Pretty amazing! I thought this was something I could get involved with, as I enjoyed home sewing.

Immediately motivated and with purpose, I got a pattern printed out from my local print shop. My sewing machine took over the kitchen table. Within a week of joining a local group, I was delivered a big roll of donated emerald-green fabric, and I got to grips with the making. Someone organised driving around, picking up and distributing. Someone else did the admin to keep up with all the home workers and requests coming in. It seemed a lot of people wanted to use their skills and time in some way. Pretty soon, I found myself part of a nationwide network of groups springing up to supply our local hospitals, care staff etc. It felt good to be doing something useful, and heartening to be part of a web of activity in the face of something so uncontrollable at the time. Though working alone, I could be in touch with others doing the same thing, and I enjoyed the camaraderie of a shared pursuit. Lots of friendly motivational banter flew around.

Many pictures popped up on the message boards. People got creative with rainbow fabric, or crazy cheery patterns and colours to lift spirits. There were scrubs hats, bags, headbands, and a multitude of advice on the technicalities of making them. There was kind feedback from the recipients, and pictures of them in multicoloured scrubs and hats on the wards. Concentrating on the making lessened my feeling of fear and kept me in the moment. The community spirit was a great unexpected comfort.

A sanctuary for all

Anita Luby

Not even a global pandemic could dampen the spirit of library workers. While officials dithered, library staff up and down the country rallied together to make sure they were there for their communities, even if they couldn't open their doors to the public for normal library services. Displaying compassion and innovation, libraries were turned into food banks for families in need. Other library staff created phone befriending services to contact vulnerable library users to make sure they were okay. Services went digital overnight, meaning baby rhyme times, story times and other important children's activities could carry on.

For those parts of our community that were digitally excluded, my library service created book bags and activity packs, which were either delivered to people's homes or available to collect from the front of our libraries. As newspaper headlines screamed of the national PPE shortage, we put our 3D printers to good use to make PPE for staff at local care homes.

During this time, The Death Positive Library project, started by Redbridge Libraries, grew as a support system for people who were feeling lost or were grieving and wanted to connect with others in a supportive network. More than 6,000 people from across the world joined our events.

We were terrified of creating virtual spaces to discuss such sensitive subjects as death and grief because we'd never done it in this way before, but we could see that people needed the collective safe space to talk that libraries are so good at providing. Libraries are a sanctuary for all, no matter who you are, where you come from or how much you have in your pockets. It was important to us that we carried on being there for our communities, even if we couldn't be with them.

The piano doctor
Jess Duckworth, clinical fellow in obstetrics and gynaecology

I have been playing the piano for as long as I can remember. My grandfather was an incredible pianist, and some of my earliest memories are of dancing around the living room to music he composed for me. I have always loved music and it was a difficult decision whether to study music or medicine. I decided to keep music as my passion and pursue medicine as a career, but I always knew I wanted to find a way to bring the two together, and so I interrupted my medical training in 2018 to do a master's degree in medical humanities. This allowed me to study the biology of how music affects the way we feel.

When we listen to music, it stimulates a part of the brain called the limbic system, which is responsible for our emotions. I wanted to compose music that would help both me and other people relax, and

I discovered that, for most people, slow melodic piano music is most effective. I use the results of this research as the basis for all my piano compositions, to enable me to create calming music for the listener.

I studied medicine in Manchester, where I spent time working with a charity bringing music into Manchester Children's Hospital. I was so amazed to see how even very sick children really lit up when we played. It was just incredible. I had been playing calming piano music in hospitals since before the pandemic and had no idea how relevant it would then become.

I moved to commence my junior doctor year training in Exeter, where I found they had a piano in the chapel, which is situated just off the main corridor of the hospital. It has lovely glass doors, which I would leave open when I was playing so the sound could just wash down the corridor. It meant that when I was playing, I wasn't cut off from the people passing. I found the best time to play for me was at the end of a night shift. They were very busy times – on duty for 12 hours straight and often without a break. And then, when the patients were sleeping and the sun was coming up, I would go and play some of the relaxing music I had composed. People would be arriving in the early hours for their day shifts and some of them would just linger briefly in the doorway or come in and sit down for a few minutes. It was lovely. The music greeted others as they arrived to work and walked past, and I hope it changed the hospital atmosphere. I received such lovely comments from people, saying how it transformed their day.

Gradually, it caught on that there was a piano doctor in the hospital, and I was asked to do some concerts in the huge restaurant there. I put together an album of my music and was absolutely blown away when it got to number one in the Official Charts for classical music albums.[1] I never expected it, but it was so encouraging to know that my music meant so much to so many people.

Playing the piano also enabled me to process my day. My compositions are based on experiences and things I had felt during my shift in hospital, and I think it meant that, by the time I got home, I could switch off and get a good night's sleep. I often spend my evenings playing piano at home after a busy shift, writing pieces about

---

1. www.facebook.com/drjessduckworth/

my day to help me reflect and relax while creating new emotions with my compositions.

I think it is so important that we bring the arts and sciences together, that we make hospitals welcoming places, not just centres of science and technology. Music can be a key element in the healing process. I think the recognition for the arts within science is broadening, as more and more hospitals are embracing the presence of music and artwork within their clinical walls and putting pianos in hospital foyers and restaurants. I have recently transitioned my training to Bristol and, excitingly, I have already found three pianos in the hospital there. One is in the main atrium, which is a perfect position from which to positively influence people's experience as they enter the hospital. My hope is that restrictions will soon lift enough for me to be able to play for patients and their families too.

Personal change stories

Standstill
Kristin Wallis

Don't get me wrong, I have been up on the Ridgeway with my dogs countless times and travelled a lot, but I had never given my closest area much attention. Oh my God! What I found. Unbelievable.

Through the viewfinder
Kiran Oram

I can't imagine anyone not carrying the impact of the past two years with them for life. For me, mortality has taken centre stage. Death appears daily – neighbours, heroes, best friends and the daily count on the news. It drags you down as if it wants you to join in. What kept me afloat was my photography, my lifebuoy.

The one thing that took me away from it all was having a camera in my hand. Studying the beauty of nature in all its forms and at all its stages. I particularly found/saw such beauty in fading flowers and also seed heads carrying the hope and possibility of future lives. This was my meditation. My escape. And I became the first non-white female member of our local photography club committee.

Untangling

Jameisha Prescod[2]

I've been living with lupus, a chronic autoimmune disease, since 2014, so the time spent working from home was supposed to allow me to make my day job more accessible to my health needs – at least, that's what I thought. I am a journalist, and during lockdown I was working from home the whole time, and I found that the work and rest division was starting to blur. Things were starting to feel out of control.

Lockdown had a heavy impact on me. Mental issues I had became amplified. I was not just unable to leave the house but, because of family difficulties, I did not really leave my room. I felt very isolated, not seeing my friends or my partner. And because of my work, I had to face the Covid situation head on every day. That's my job. As well as finding it tough emotionally, I was handling some physical issues too. I had to have surgery and then there were complications. That was hard for me, that it all snowballed at the same time. It was hard for lots of people

I was taught knitting by my granma as a kid. I was not great at it at first. I took a massive break from it. Then I picked up the knitting again. Sometimes I felt bad I was doing it, like it was procrastinating, but actually I found that the repetitive motion helped me organise my mind and I felt proud of finishing something that was not just about work. And there was a connection with my granma. She has stopped knitting now. There was a link, but it was more cool and modernised: I was making hats and tops; she was crocheting doilies.

There was this satisfaction of organising a ball of chaos and making something out of it. It was a lifeline. It was away from expected productivity.

One day I was sitting there knitting and I thought, 'I'll take a picture.' I took it without really feeling it was that significant. I was thinking, 'I am not going to hide my room.' It was a mess. Instead of, like, shying away from it, I tried to capture it. I put my camera by the window for best light and took it wearing the clothes I had on. That's why I call it a documentary photo. I saw it and thought it was

---

2. Jameisha's self-portrait, 'Untangling', was one of the winners of the Wellcome Photography Prize 2021. https://wellcome.org/what-we-do/our-work/wellcome-photography-prize/2021

framed nicely but I'm still quite surprised that it won the Wellcome Prize. I'm kind of pleased and horrified. I was glad that other people felt seen and affirmed – that they connected with the picture. We were all trying to hide our backgrounds. I am also horrified because it is a bit of a taboo in my culture. I'm Afro-Caribbean and it is not acceptable to show people your mess. You tidy up before people come over, innit. It feels like taboo to show that vulnerable part of my life, but I have made peace with that. It is for the greater good. People feeling less ashamed.

Winning the prize was amazing. I don't do it for that but now I feel affirmed as a creative person. It has really helped my confidence. I have always wanted to be able to work for myself but never felt that it could be a thing. It is not easy for people with chronic unpredictable health conditions. I want to be able to control how my health interacts with my work – honouring the rest as much as the work, and now I believe I can work towards that future. I didn't think it was possible before. **www.instagram.com/youlookokaytome/?hl=en**

Being fat in a post-Covid world

@HeardinLondon

I have been speaking to a lot of people lately who are nervous about going back to crowded places. And not because they're frightened of the crowds, but because they're frightened of being judged for the changes in their bodies over lockdown. Fatphobia is so ingrained in our culture that a huge number of people are able to dismiss the fact that their bodies just survived a global pandemic and are more worried about whether that old pair of jeans will still fit them anymore.

How have we got to the point where we are able to completely overlook the miracle that we actually survived because of anxiety about how we look? What if you made the decision that you were going to use this pandemic as a life changer, and that treating yourself unkindly was something that you left in the before times?

A golden time

Margaret Nairne

Late March 2020 and my eldest son, aged 29, rang from London where he and his Dutch girlfriend had packed up their belongings and were ready for their permanent move to Amsterdam, a rental flat lined up:

'Mum, I think we might have to come and live with you and Dad – do you think we might come and live with you?' All three of my children were living in London and I'd only stashed enough toilet rolls for two. With some apprehension, I replied, 'Of course you can – come, come!' They stayed for more than three months and, with four of us working at home, we quickly established a harmonious routine. We took in the news each day but, keenly aware of what was happening beyond our own short horizon, for us the sun shone, and we walked and we cooked and we talked. The weeks and then months were an unforeseen, precious gift no one could ever have predicted. We fell for the Dutch girl, and living so closely with her and our son has undoubtedly changed the course of our relationships with them. How extraordinary, and for us, how serendipitous, to normalise our adult children living at home again for extended periods – we look back now at an unsettling yet golden time.

The great escape

My mother was admitted to a care home in January 2020, after a spell in hospital to recuperate from a hip operation. She has dementia and was living with my brother, who was dependent on her since his sight had almost gone and he has Bardet-Biedl syndrome.

She enjoyed the company in the care home, was well cared for and was able to rest. Then came Covid. The care home imposed a no-visiting rule and restricted residents to their rooms for most of the day, only allowing them out for one hour. Staff were not all equipped with gloves and masks and we were very afraid of her catching the virus and about the impact on her mental health. There was no vaccine back then. We managed to visit Mum and talk to her through an open window twice, but she is deaf so it was not great, although she did know we were there. I had a horror of her isolated like that and we decided that we should get her out sooner than planned and before any cases were reported in her care home. I had this overriding conviction she would just fade away in there without social contact, particularly with her family.

That is when we hit problems. We did not have a health and welfare Lasting Power of Attorney for her and so we found that social services were in charge. That was very upsetting. I did not have a leg to stand on. We had to fight to claim my mother back. We had to go through all their checks and procedures. That took three-and-a-half agonising weeks. We were new to the entire process. I called the home often to see if there had been a case, knowing that, if there was, we might never get her out. It was so stressful. We contacted our local councillor to support our case. We even considered jumping her. We were desperate.

We were able to give assurances that I would be at home caring for her 24 hours a day. Everything moved so agonisingly slowly because, of course, social services were under huge strain and the system did not seem fit for purpose. We were lucky we could create a ground-floor bedroom for her, so our house was considered suitable.

It felt like a fight. It shouldn't have done. We got her out just as the first cases arrived in the home. To see her utter joy at being home again and witness how her spirits lifted and her health improved were their own reward. And it was better for my brother, who had also moved in with us. I felt incredibly privileged to care for my mum and grateful to my wife and son for supporting me. The process of looking after her and dealing with all the pee and poo and pads and the confusion – in a way, it didn't seem difficult. It is just what you do when you love someone. We haven't look back since then. She has remained at home. It was quite a discovery to know you have that strong fight in you, if you need it, to protect those you love.

Down and up
Emma
Running keeps me sane. I mean that quite literally. Without it, I start to go downhill. When my husband got Covid and I could not leave our house, I ran up and down in the garden and bought a lot of fitness equipment. He recovered and I got quite fit.

Creature comfort
Amber was my constant companion while my husband was at work. When he died suddenly in January 2019, she became even more important as a comforter – always there, showing affection, never demanding. A little life-saver during those dark days.

Sadly, later the same year, I had to part with her, after 13 years. It was double devastation. After three days of being on my own in an empty house, and when my 'get up and go' had gone, I was lucky to find Poppy – an eight-week-old bundle of mischief. She filled my days during lockdown and isolation. I still had to take her for walks and so I met other people (albeit at a distance), so at least I was able to converse, get fresh air and exercise – all so important to the healing process.

I sincerely believe that, without the companionship of first Amber and then Poppy, I would not have got through the past two years as sanely as I like to think I have. When a warm, soft, furry little face is pressed into your hand and loving, big brown eyes look up at you, it is heart-warming.

Change of career
Andrew Pennington

I followed a straight path from university into full-time work as an aeronautical engineer. Never had time to consider the path my life was taking.

Then came lockdown and the unexpected mental freedom brought about by working from home. Without the requirement to commute, and without the opportunity to make plans of almost any kind, the conditions for introspection became much more favourable. And so I started to think more seriously about how I wanted to spend my working life. Mental barriers came up: How could I give up a well-paid job and salary? I had worked for so many years in my field – was it too late to change now? I know people do change careers, but was I really one of those people?

I had enjoyed the technical side of my career to date, and the opportunities to travel, but something had been missing: the wish to work in a way that more obviously helped people in some way. This may have stemmed from some volunteering I started doing with an emotional support charity some years previously. I also wanted a career that would allow me the flexibility to move almost anywhere in the country; my partner's job as a teacher was already a flexible one, and both of us would like to one day move closer to where we grew up, to be nearer to family. Being near to family wasn't something either of us considered much when we left school or university but has now taken on more importance.

Despite the current pressures on the NHS, the hospital environment appealed as a place to work – perhaps from having watched so many documentaries about A&E departments. Then came the idea of working in radiography. The more I looked into it, the more it seemed to have potential. Almost every hospital in the country has a radiology department served by a team of radiographers. It's a technical role – something that appeals to my scientific side – yet also involves working with patients in a caring and supportive way. It's not a job that even occurred to me when I left school, and being much shyer then, working in a hospital environment with patients would have been much more of a shock to the system.

I am still in training. It's a three-year course but I found one near where I live. I am a student again. I find it so rewarding helping people in need. I meet all kinds of people and I really am able to help. It helps put life into perspective. So different from the corporate world.

Despite all the terrible things the pandemic has brought, it gave me – and I suspect many others – the chance to take a step back and assess the direction of their lives. In that way, I am fortunate that it has changed mine for the better.

Coming home
Helen Chadwick

I had long needed to leave London and planned a return to the West Country. Then, into the gap of uncertainty, walked a friend who suggested I borrow a house overlooking the Firth of Clyde – a view over tidal waters, islands, with the mountains behind me. Although it seemed a mad choice to go so far from collaborators and friends, the place answered a deeper necessity I'd long held in check for the purposes of work. It was a coming home to the needs of body and soul.

And I find myself happy – happy walking up a hill, happy watching the ever-changing light, happy to work, happy under my Colombian blanket with its memories of safety in the midst of danger, happy with my extra-large mug of tea, happy singing with others who need to sing in person, happy that life is not the same but constantly new, happy to go back to a simple piece of Schumann on the piano and never become bored of its beauty, happy to go to bed when it's cold, happy to be alive.

But beyond the place, something else happened. Someone recommended a scientific book about near-death experiences, hundreds and thousands of them. Death has been a topic all my life, in my song writing and in my shows. I have sung for and about the dead and dying and I know the taste and fierce battering of loss intimately. But this book shifted something again. It echoed with previous experiences in my life, and I started to feel that death might be a wonderful thing, could itself be welcomed, however unfinished our lives seem. This is an utterly absurd thing to say in the knowledge of illness, suffering and death that each of us holds. In the response to Covid, the whole emphasis was initially on staying alive, but this is not the most important thing for me anymore. Perhaps it never was.

Peace and quiet
Mary Maltby

Like for many, my experience during lockdown was full of frustrations, but it was also full of gifts. It allowed me to put down my 'shoulds' and 'oughts' and enjoy the simplicity of life. I started walking two miles each day – not because I should or ought to, but because I wanted to. I loved the opportunity to simply be with nature. Each day was different, and each walk was different. I was fortunate to be living in the beautiful countryside, so many of my walks were in silence, hearing only the birds and the sounds of nature. It gave me such a sense of peace. I would often meet my neighbours walking their dogs or riding their horses and we would say how lucky we were to be living in a such a beautiful setting where we could simply meet and greet each other outdoors without the fear of getting Covid. Many of them were new to the village and I was able to make lasting friendships. I look back on my experience of lockdown with appreciation and joy.

Making a move

I started the Covid pandemic in the United States, locked down in a large city-apartment building, a single parent with two children. I went from having an office-based job and a child in elementary (primary) school and one in nursery, to being a 24/7 full-time parent, employee and teacher. The initial months of the pandemic were occupied by social distancing, online shopping and trying to simultaneously be three different people. Every day was scheduled with meticulous detail, to ensure that school, work, meals, along with a little fresh air, were somehow fitted in.

But some clouds have silver linings. While the pandemic brought isolation and challenges, it also brought opportunity. Opportunities to do things differently, evaluate what is important and re-prioritise.

With work entirely online, colleagues and friends began to move – closer to family, away from the city for a different pace of life, to take advantage of a new-found flexibility. Six months in, with the prospect of a new school year still online and my youngest starting school remotely, came a new opportunity for me too. Moving back to family in the UK, where schools were offering in-person education and where I would have family support, made sense. It was clearly the better option for the children's education and for me.

Luckily my job was willing to take a chance and try something new too. Despite the restrictions of Covid, I was still able to spend more time with family than I had done in years. Working from a different time zone provided more unexpected bonuses – the ability to volunteer at school without taking time off work and a chance to engage in some of my own interests before starting the work day. I've now chosen to continue to work remotely and from home, allowing me to continue to be more engaged in my children's lives and have a better work-life balance.

Early retirement
Paul Julian

I had been considering retirement for some time, but had not progressed matters for a number of reasons, including how much I was continuing to enjoy work. This despite the fact that I had lots of ideas about what I wanted to do post-working.

The early days of Covid brought many changes to my working environment, meaning that the usual office-based methods were replaced by remote working. At first this was fun and meant that commuting time became time for thinking and drinking tea. As the weeks and months went by, though, the enjoyment faded and was overtaken by frustration that communications were not as constructive as they had been when colleagues were in the same room.

Then, when an opportunity arose for me to realise my plan to cease working, I took the retirement option, in the midst of the uncertainties of 2021 lockdowns, seemingly ever-changing guidance and the unknown shape of the future.

I am not the type to need to pin down the future and the pandemic showed me that this was likely to be a very useful trait, for the initial period at least. The unknown shape of what's to come I regarded as exciting, which helped me cope with the post-work environment I encountered.

The first few months were spent mainly outdoors in the UK, indulging my love of walking in the hills; choosing times and locations that synchronised with restrictions to maximise time away while working within the relevant national guidance at that time.

I also refurbished the kitchen, which had been difficult when I was working away during the week.

I am very grateful for the push that Covid gave me, with the knowledge that moving towards a 'life of leisure' was always what I wanted but had previously not been ready to embrace.

I continue to wonder what's next, and whilst restrictions and variants abound, will take small steps to explore options (likely to include volunteering in some form) and more hillsides!

Solo lockdowns

First lockdown – all the unknowns. Is this real? A manufactured crisis creating fear to manipulate the public? Who to believe? Lamentable public health messaging… So many brown faces among the NHS staff Covid casualties – what's going on?! Alert those I know to take vitamin D…

If my breathing fails, would I call for help to go to hospital or to a shaman to help me die well? Reflect on how to die at home. (Must write a will…) Fear of the unknown.

Savour nature's silence in the midst of the city. Traffic noise fades; few planes; clearer skies; star-gazing from my doorstep; vibrant birdsong. It's a glorious spring.

Acclimatise to Zoom. Appreciate renewed connection with family members. Appreciate my neighbours. Appreciate my solitude.

And shrink in that same solitude, like a visceral vacuum, missing the physical presence of humans, conversations, sharing a meal, human touch. I count the months since my last hug, a deep longing. Absence. Bereft and alone, circling the pit of depression. My introvert has taken over. It is increasingly difficult to reach out or make contact with friends.

I long to walk in nature, unbounded by the concrete skyline. An opportunity for a legitimate work trip to the countryside! Driving down the empty motorway, I feel deskilled after being at home so long.

Arriving in the huge green landscape with distant horizons under vast blue skies, every cell in my body sings with joy. Breathe in nature's balm through every pore. Staying overnight with two old friends, I discover my social skills are also rusty... I am so excited, like an overflowing fizzy bottle, but terribly sensitive, lacking the usual social veneer. I retreat to my solitary cave, but the memory of the vast vibrant natural world stays.

Escape
Liz Rothschild

Here the dark cormorant still wings its unswerving way north

The grebes duck and dive

The ducks congregate in chattering posses without regard to social
  distancing.

The trees dip their branches towards the lapping water.

I shed my clothes and wade in, fingers trailing strands of light.

Making for the centre of the lake

Embraced by the cold.

I roll onto my back.

Sky!

Uneventful unfettered expansive

And this body of water

My body in this water,

Of this water

Deep and constant

Soothing me

Welcoming me home.

At last I can hear myself not think.

Isolationship
Debbie Collins

Sauntering along platform five at Marylebone, gentling anticipation running through me, 'Will I recognise him?' 'What if he's ghastly?' 'How long can I reasonably stay?' 'What if he's lovely and I don't want to leave?' Feet moving me ever closer… The barrier, looking across, taller than I thought, looking expectantly, yes, that must be him… Meeting with smiles and hellos… him confidently walking us to Hyde Park… I like being guided by someone who knows – the geography of London has forever been a mystery to me… Talking, talking …. Sitting drinking tea, telling family stories of dysfunction… and connection … Risking the tube a few stops, even though we've been told this new virus is probably dangerous…

Messaging… he's visiting relatives and could make a detour to stay a night… Excitement punctuating my day's work… showing him my town, sitting in my favourite restaurant… feeling the risk of eating out in an almost empty place… sharing stories… I like him, he's interesting, funny, and he likes me… Parting for sleep, in the morning kitchen, he's in jeans only… He's in good shape…

Messaging… reality of lockdown coming… what to do? We live alone, hours apart… could we risk seeing the few weeks out together? What if I go to his and find I am trapped by a crazy axe murderer? He assures me I could have his daughter's room and continue my yoga practice and work… Eventually, it's decided he'll come to me… His car breaks down halfway… He has to choose whether to go home or… He chooses me… Flurry of arrival… his car stuffed to the gunnels… filling cupboards, overflowing fridges… carrying pictures, duvet, pillows to his room… Later, on the sofa together… tired and shaking with the enormity of saying yes… fear catching up… a stranger, feeling trapped in my own home… internal battle of opening to him and closing, closing…

A new routine begins… Breakfast on a tray sitting at the foot of his bed… morning talks before my newly shaped working day begins… contacting clients and friends to stay in touch in this strange new world… Spring… he wants work and takes on a gargantuan task in which I periodically join him… Sun shining day after day… lunch in the garden, catering for ourselves, holding onto some of our old shapes… Walking at the end of working days… swans tending their nest… hare scrabbling out of the canal… heron presiding, long beak poised… tiny muntjac skittering away… turning away from people, mouth and nose covered…

Assurances we can go slowly sexually… that it doesn't matter if it doesn't happen… beginning to thaw the cold. We could… and yet…

I cannot re-open myself… afraid… cajoling, coaxing, stroking… protecting, holding tight, withdrawing…

Lockdown is ending. His car arrives… he is leaving… Predictably, I do not want him to go… hold on tight… and then release… We've been brave… we honour our courage in trying. We were brave… it was good to try… old patterns prevailed.

Keeping the faith

Adele Moss

How did we all survive as a community in the past two years? Was there distance? Of course. We couldn't meet in any normal way. Was there connection? Yes, profoundly so. People reaching out with all their resourcefulness, creativity and imagination and with all their hearts. There were wide ranging efforts to make sure nobody fell through the safety net: practical, spiritual and emotional. I was paired up with a phone buddy whom I'd never met, and she has become a dear friend. Jewish worship, although including personal prayer, is based on the presence of 10 people sharing a space together, but we had to find some way forward. Different religious practices called for different solutions. For those who didn't use technology on Shabbat, there were Zoom services that took us up to the threshold – sunset on Friday evening, when we greeted the Sabbath singing the luscious verses of the Song of Solomon.

For Passover, our family and friends were virtual guests at the ritual meal, and we gave takeaway food to the ones who lived nearby. On Rosh Hashana, my daughter blew her shofar during our prayers at home, with a sense of awe and acute longing for her community. One young woman kindly brought her shofar to the homes of isolated people and blew it in their gardens.

At the end of Yom Kippur, the Day of Atonement, a 25-hour fast, after a day of socially distanced, masked, intense and muted prayers in the synagogue, we couldn't enjoy our usual delicious and highly sociable break-fast, the yearly generous gift of a very kind couple. This would normally be a time of such release and warmth as people had their first cup of tea and found out how others had experienced the fast or what had happened to them since they last met. Instead, this couple sent each person home with a break-fast in a bag. Not the same thing, but all that love – in a paper bag. Our Jewish story reflects the spirit I saw all around me – one of courage and compassion, overlying sadness and longing. To quote the poet Amanda Gorman:

> To love just may be
> The fight of our lives[3]

Tuning in

Marguerite Wallis

We remain in physical isolation (not social isolation, as is advised), just in case my elderly mother becomes ready to be discharged. She lives near Abergavenny. I live in Oxford. I have found a way to be with her through prayer and in the depths of meditation, willing the peace I tune into to hold her too. When we are prevented from doing what comes naturally, the only option is to turn inwards to the sanctuary of the heart. As Good Friday approaches, I think of Jesus on the cross and feel all of humanity is in some way on the cross now and facing loss. When all this is over, what might the resurrected earth and heart be like?

Making form from chaos

Laura Potts

What fell away in March 2020: all the busyness, the days' different tasks and responsibilities jigsawed into not quite enough time. What came to fill those days: agitation and fear, a longing for connection and a terror of seeing anyone. Less to do, more to feel. A disjointed isolation, a formlessness, an absence of rhythm, apart from my yoga practice and teaching, which still gave shape and some purpose, a long-established daily discipline holding body and soul together.

To distil and contain each day, I started to write a daily haiku, from just before the spring equinox until the summer solstice. And during the new emptier days – missing my mother, declining with dementia in a care home where I could no longer visit her; going for slow walks around the allotments and out on the strays;[4] tending my garden; talking on the phone; teaching yoga online – I would

---

3. From 'Atonement', in *Poems: Call us what we carry*, published Chatto & Windus (2021).

4. The strays is a collective name for four areas of open land within the City of York.

be forming lines, counting syllables, balancing words. Making form from chaos.

March 31st
Stretching the hours out,
I've seldom done so little.
The birds are louder.

And as a grower, there was no denying it was spring. Which always demands attention and work: seeds must be sown when the conditions are right, and energy has to be directed to the earth, judging the air, watering what emerges with care.

I've always recorded the emergence of spring buds and birds, and now those observations kept connection to past years, renewing those delights in first sightings.

April 17th
Warmth of the soil now,
Planting peas. A speckled wood.
We must endure more.

Letter to the Prison Phoenix Trust

Maria

August 2020

My name is Maria. I am a foreign national. I've been in prison here nearly a year and waiting for trial in October this year. I am writing to thank you for the free meditation and yoga books you sent me.

In one book, there is an Islamic prayer that gives me strength. Although I'm not Muslim, I'm Catholic. But it gives me hope and makes me smile, which in a situation like this could be difficult sometimes.

O Allah
Enlighten what is dark in me.
Strengthen what is weak in me.
Mend what is broken in me.
Bind what is bruised in me.
Heal what is sick in me.

Straighten what is crooked in me.

And revive whatever peace and love has died in me…

Ameen

August 2021

Here everything still is like lockdown. There are rumours some activities will start soon, but then you hear the opposite. I've learned not to trust any of that, because everything is always changing and too fast. There are a few women here wearing a mask. However the staff do, which I like. It sets an example. A good one.

I don't know how things are outside. Only what is said on the news and the friend I call. Doing yoga has become my morning routine because of Covid, so is not something bad. I am trying to find the silver lining during this storm, and I do feel better since I am practising. It is a shame the yoga lessons stopped too, but it's our safety at risk. I understand.

Remember the couple of quotes you sent me some time ago? They also contribute (when I feel down) to feel better. 'Everything can be taken from a man but one thing, the last of human freedoms – to choose one's attitude in any given set of circumstances, to choose one's own say.' Victor Frankl. Thank you!

My practice is my own and is a treasure no one can take away from me. I get nervous some days thinking about the trial, the transfer. So I've been meditating more and sitting in my chair! Not lying on bed. So I can see myself doing it more and more, not because I feel okay.

I'm going to leave it here. Thank you for staying in touch, keep staying safe.

Love Maria.

Saturday night

Throughout the pandemic I lived with three other girls (all in our 20s): a physiotherapist, a care home assistant and a graphic designer. We all moved in as strangers. In the care home, there was a vast outbreak of Delta variant and a huge proportion of residents passed away. Our little physio took the hit and was deployed to the Covid ward and, as a junior doctor, I felt like it never ended. Our resident graphic designer worked from home and sat, wide-eyed at the dinner table, watching us ride the rollercoaster on the frontline each week.

But on every Saturday night of that dark January, we did a weekly three-course, full formal-attire 'Come Dine with Me' extravaganza. Mexican fiesta week with a home-made piñata, churros and too many tequila cocktails and an imaginary trip to an Italian roadside Mezze bar being the top scorers.

Alpha-omega – interbeing
Stuart Taylor

Surely it's always the case, that we the survivors, the ones that grieve and mourn, are left to remake our lives, somehow refashion them, in the wake of such profound loss. The death of a parent. The first to leave our nuclear family web. A profound shock. A hitherto unimaginable readjustment. I understand now that this carnival, this riot of feelings in all its tumultuousness, is something that we humans have experienced since we began, so many millennia ago. However, in the here and now, in the 21st century, these feelings are as immediate, intense and raw as I imagine they ever were.

Bizarrely, there were numerous restrictions and spatial distancing in operation at the time of our final farewell. Live streaming of her funeral too. Some immediate family members were cast as remote participants, through the 'magic' of Zoom. Somehow, though, even amongst this strangeness within strangeness, it worked out. Our final parting happened. We shed our tears and recalled with fondness the best of our times together. We remembered the best of the qualities she expressed, shared with Dad and handed on to us, her children.

The death of a loved one and mourning them are surreal at the best of times, I am told, have read and now experienced. On what scale can we measure or convey the depth of our feelings in a time of technology-enabled funerary rites, deep within a pandemic? Somehow, we managed. Somehow, we made sense. We offered the finest of our words. We shed the saltiest of tears. Then we laughed and recalled the unique contours of her life and ways. As a family. As friends and neighbours. The sun shone down upon our impromptu wake, bees pollinated the very flowers she lovingly planted and tended over many decades. They bloomed. Beautifully. In the garden and in our hearts.

a shimmering joy
winter 2021

yes grief is complex
showing the depth of our love
for those we have lost

something like the tides
but with its unique rhythms
unpredictable

this human knowing
bonds us to our ancestors
whom we will become

the wisdom in this
that our hearts become a bridge
between death and life

a distinctive gift
one of divine origin
infusing each breath

shaping the meaning
in all the moments we share
precious transient

reverence is due
to honour and praise this love
across the aeons
the thread of life glows
we are connected to all
each of us belong

moonlight reflecting
on the waters of our life
a shimmering joy

Commentary
Liz Rothschild

This chapter naturally divided itself into two sections: community responses, where people gathered together to protect the most vulnerable in their neighbourhood or sought to support those working on the frontline, and the individual discoveries people made about how they chose to change how they lived.

It often takes a crisis in our lives to jolt us out of unhelpful patterns we have settled into and regard as unchangeable. For example, for years there have been attempts to establish more flexible working practices, which suddenly became the norm when employers realised it was the only way to remain in business. This exposed the lack of will to explore these options seriously before, despite pressure to do so from some employees. Individuals who had dreamed of making changes in their working life suddenly took the plunge. This, of course, has had other unintended consequences. People choosing to live in more rural areas have, in some places, disrupted the local economy. I was told that, in Kendal, when many workers had to leave the area due to the lack of work in the leisure industry, many multiple occupancy houses where they had been renting rooms were sold to people moving into the area. Now there is a crisis as there is nowhere for the returning workforce to live that they can afford, many businesses are struggling to recruit staff, and commuting is too costly for workers on a minimum wage.

We caught a glimpse of a world in which planet-damaging travel could be dramatically reduced and where nature began to reclaim spaces normally dominated by human activity. With amazing speed, birdsong dominated the city soundscape, goats gambolled through Llandudno and deer browsed the grass in housing estates in parts of London. Some parents got the opportunity to share caring responsibilities more equitably. Online platforms have enabled those with access to technology to participate in a wide range of events they might have been excluded from before – talks, seminars, podcasts, support groups, exercise and a range of creative arts. The will to explore this type of delivery had not been felt before (although the need was always there).

Covid has forced us to create a new template for future, more creative and inclusive practices.

So what did we miss? It varied according to our circumstances, of course. Physical contact, sharing experiences with others face to face, a sense of purpose, creativity, fun and variety, structure, contact with the natural world, significant family and community events, holidays, a regular income, secure housing, physical safety and the chance to receive a meaningful education. This chapter looks at how some people tried to compensate for some of these losses.

I love the way Diane Harris describes placing the rainbow picture in her window (p.161). It's an act we saw repeated around the country and one that we perhaps became less responsive to over time, but here she takes us into the detail of that gesture with refreshing self-deprecation and reveals her desire to help others. 'So now people will either think I have flipped or be astounded at my talent. Opposite me is a nursing home. Maybe my rainbow will bring a smile to someone's face.' Small actions can carry great significance.

Others begin to meet and greet their neighbours in a way they never have before. Again, an easily overlooked exchange and one to which we seldom pay attention in more usual circumstances. That simple act of connection can transform people's day. They feel recognised, safer, part of their neighbourhood and, by extension, more able to ask for help if needed. We have been reminded of the importance of knowing our neighbours, not just cultivating a chosen circle of friends and family who may all live very far away from us geographically. I think of these relationships like the very fine, delicate roots you can easily miss but that are essential in keeping a plant stable in the earth. It is also notable how these new connections endured in places. Jude Bishop describes how new groups regularly meeting face to face once restrictions eased met a need that had not been clearly identified before or certainly not prioritised (p.164).

In reading the stories about the organised community responses, I am struck by several things. The speed with which a lot of complex processes were put in place is astonishing and could not have happened without the use of social media and technology. It is also profoundly heartening to be reminded of how much people want to share their skills and their time in order to help others. This is not the prevailing narrative in most news outlets. Sarah Grylls describes very well the impulse to help (p.163): 'I need to feel engaged with the world, to act and have an impact on it, in order to keep my sense of self intact.' This is healthy self-interested altruism. Sophy Thomas (p.169) reiterates this, saying that, once she found out about the scrubs project, she was 'immediately motivated and with purpose'. It is notable that, while remaining in isolation throughout, she also felt valued and connected through social media, receiving a stream of tips, jokes, pictures and thanks to enliven her days.

The value of helping those who help is made explicit in the Manchester Mind project (p.165), which works with people living with mental health challenges. A double benefit results for those volunteering and those receiving the food: 'Having the opportunity to go and help cook and prepare food with a lovely team really boosted my mood and gave me energy for the rest of the day.' Animal companionship saw many people through the loneliness and isolation. In *Citizens* (2022), Jon Alexander and Ariane Conrad point out that 750,000 people tried to sign up as first responders within 48 hours and 100,000 volunteered to help deliver the vaccine programme. Polls conducted by More in Common (2020) reveal that the percentage of those reporting a heightened sense of being part of a community 'who understand, care for and help each other' rose from 49% to 63% during the pandemic.

The flexibility and resilience shown by many large organisations was demonstrated by the way they transformed their delivery. Anita Luby (p.169) tells us about libraries going out into the community in unprecedented ways, with book bags to serve those most impacted by school closures and lockdown – not to mention using their 3D printer to create personal protective equipment. Many arts organisations also began streaming performances, offering virtual gallery tours, inviting online participation and getting artists to share work remotely. Creative collaborations became much closer between organisations that, in the past, might have seen themselves as rivals for sources of funding or audiences. This happened in Bristol, for example, where the Watershed, Bristol Old Vic and Bristol Museum collaborated more closely.

As someone who has been involved with the arts for much of my working life, I was relieved to find people acutely feeling their absence and really appreciating the role they play in our lives and valuing the online concerts delivered from home, the regular home discos and other invitations. Equally, creatives began to see that their work was not complete without an audience. I heard the pianist Beatrice Rana talking to Tom Service on Radio 3 about performing in a live concert for the first time after seven months. The musicians applauded the audience for coming out. She realised that previously she had taken the audience for granted. We have come to value our relationships much more highly. The contribution from Jess Duckworth (p.170) shows just how crucial the arts can be in promoting our psychological wellbeing, which in turns leads to physical healing. So often, when talking about budgets, hospitals are set against arts venues, which I believe is a false dichotomy. Both are able to contribute to both preventative and curative medicine, not to mention expand our field of understanding about the world and enable us to empathise with those whose experiences are very different from our own.

Religious organisations have also had to adapt. In Chapter 4, we heard about a young person streaming his church services online (p.105). I am moved by the account in this chapter of the shofar (a type of horn used in the synagogue) being blown in people's gardens (p.184). It reflects for me a deep, instinctive knowing about the value of such a simple sound to connect us with our kin, rather as I imagine the call of the muezzin does for a Muslim believer. I suspect too that the actual quality of the sound and how it reverberates in our bodies when we hear it has soothing and healing properties, reaching out to touch with sound, if not with a human hand. Others, like Marguerite Wallis (p.185). felt that, through their own meditative or prayerful practice, they were able to close the physical distance between themselves and their family members or the outside world.

Then there has been a huge expansion of classes, such as yoga and meditation online. Yes, as a yoga teacher friend told me, there is the loss of being unable to make hands-on postural corrections but, conversely, each student must take fuller responsibility for what they are doing and really scrutinise their own practice.

I myself have been surprised how much emotion and contact can be generated during Zoom gatherings. Ruth Rosselson talks more about this in her account of her work, offering peer support to very vulnerable people (p.167).

The outbreak of breadmaking and baking became a bit of a cliché, but what a wonderfully simple and inclusive process Rana Ibrahim created (p.166), breaking down the isolation of the daily task of preparing meals.

How have we all been presenting ourselves online during meetings and other sessions? There were a lot of jokes circulating about people doing Zoom meetings still wearing their pyjama bottoms and carefully curating their bookshelves to present a suitable image of themselves. Into this narrative comes Jameisha Prescod (p.173), deciding on an impulse to photograph herself and her messy room just as she was and, as a result, not only winning a prestigious prize but also reducing her own and other's feelings of isolation and shame.

Work, home, relationships and leisure activities all came under scrutiny and many of us were either forced into making or chose to make quite drastic alterations.

Again and again I observe a theme in these accounts of paying close attention to what we were doing or seeing and really appreciating it as a result. 'The one thing that took me away from it all was having a camera in my hand… This was my meditation and escape,' writes Kiran Oram (p.172). As the poet Mary Oliver wonderfully observes (2016), 'Attention is the beginning of devotion.' I wonder what you, the reader, discovered. It seems to me that those who fared best were able either to connect with others or focus on what really mattered to them – be it gardening, walking, knitting, playing music, cooking, writing poetry or learning a new skill. The focus required and the discoveries that emerged enlivened them. Many, of course, had no spare time for themselves and clearly those struggling financially found it almost impossible to benefit in this way. However, the story from Maria in prison, about the impact of meditation and yoga, shows how people can create a space for positive self-reflection and new perspectives even in the least likely of environments (p.186).

Many relationships were severed or severely impacted. Tragically, in a number of households, the confinement led to or exacerbated domestic violence and abuse – there was a reported 30–40% increase in calls to helplines and more deaths from domestic violence during the lockdowns (ONS, 2021). However, there were also positive outcomes. Some people who had only recently met tried living together to avoid isolation, with more or less success (p.182). Some communities live intergenerationally, and in less affluent households there is sometimes no choice, whatever the preferences of those involved. For many white, middle-class families, it is unusual to share your home with your adult children. Margaret Nairne (p.174) captures a precious period when she and her husband really got to know their son's new partner through sharing a house with them during lockdown, and so laid down a precious foundation for the future.

A number of families decided they could not leave their relatives in residential care or isolated in independent living. For one storyteller, who came close to having to kidnap their elderly mother from the care home, there were no regrets (p.175) – only a sense of safety and security. The story also underlines the crucial importance of ensuring you have lasting powers of attorney in place for when they might be needed.

Connecting to the non-human world also became crucially important to many people. Animals feature large here. The value of pets in easing the process of grieving, bringing interest and energy into a family's daily routine and company into the life of someone living alone cannot be underestimated (see p.176). Chaplains at Cardiff University started a weekly walk-and-talk event and brought along their dogs to give students a little bit of normality and get them outside. Many people bought dogs during the pandemic, to accompany their permitted walks; the return to office hours and bases has meant a considerable spike in the numbers of these puppies now being taken to dog shelters for rehoming or abandoned, many of them requiring medical treatment due to poor breeding practices during the pandemic when demand and prices were so high.[5]

People also became alert to their need to be outside. The farmhouse I used to live in has a public footpath passing alongside it, which was used regularly but not extensively before lockdown. Suddenly, it was in constant use by runners, walkers and cyclists. A manager of the Royal Parks in London told me that people visiting the parks were no longer mostly tourists; instead, they were exclusively local residents, leading the Parks staff to adapt how they interacted with the public. In this chapter we read of people becoming alive to what they have in their locality, valuing parks and green spaces to which they have access on foot or even moving away from urban centres to live in remote rural areas. One storyteller here describes the walking group she set up in

---

5. https://adch.org.uk/wp-content/uploads/2021/02/ADCH-Covid-Impact-Survey-No.3-as-at-January-2021.pdf

an outer London borough that continues to meet and walk to this day (p.165). There is a vast amount of research showing how our mental and physical health and wellbeing are nourished by being outside in green spaces, or even just looking at pictures of landscapes.[6] I see the truth of this every day with families at my green burial ground.

For some, reading the story of surviving Covid will be hard because of their own losses. They have been left traumatised and bereft by what they experienced and still do not feel their losses have been properly acknowledged. And yet it is important to remember that most people have re-emerged. Some will continue to live with the effects of that experience, but most of us discovered reserves of resilience in ourselves that we might not have known were there. For a more detailed account of the experience of recovering from Covid, I recommend Michael Rosen's excellent book (2021) *Many Different Kinds of Love.*

As restrictions eased, there was talk of returning to normal. Some people were fearful because they believed it was too soon. Others never believed there should have been any lockdown measures in the first place. Some questioned whether returning to the normal as we knew it was an option at all, or even desirable. What version of normal did we inhabit before? How did we view our society and our world? Whose version of normal dominated? Wasn't this an opportunity for doing things differently, given that how we were living contributed in no small part to the pandemic and our struggles to survive its repercussions? In the light of the growing climate emergency, our normal is constantly shifting and changing and impacting our lives, even if those of us living in inland areas in Western Europe are less alive to that than more vulnerable communities and nations. What kind of normal do we need now? Are we really expecting to return to a model of constant economic growth, even as war comes to Europe and the cost of living is soaring? So many of us have begun to experience directly the fragility of our global food chain and energy supply, thanks to events beyond our borders.

We have come to realise the profound value of our friends and communities, our hunger for shared experiences, artistic expression

---

6. See, for example, www.mind.org.uk/information-support/tips-for-everyday-living/nature-and-mental-health/how-nature-benefits-mental-health

and the simple comfort of touch. I hope these discoveries will lead us to revise our priorities and consider more deeply what kind of future we are leaving to future generations.

The closing piece in this chapter invites us to connect with our ancestors. In writing about death (p.186), Stuart Taylor is also very much writing about life. Drawing on the many rich strands of his heritage, he shows us that, just like the flow of the tides, death needs to be accepted, included and allowed to flow through our lives. What all the stories in this chapter, and indeed this whole book, demonstrate to me is something I have long held to be true: that the fierce proximity of death can, if we are fortunate, draw us closer together and vividly alert us to the preciousness of life.

References

Alexander, J. & Conrad, A. (2022). *Citizens: Why the key to fixing everything is all of us.* Canonbury Press.

More in Common. (2020). *Britain's Choice: Common ground and division in 2020s Britain.* More in Common. https://www.britainschoice.uk/

Oliver, M. (2016). *Upstream: Selected essays.* Penguin Press.

ONS.(2021).*Domesticabuseduringthecoronavirus(COVID-19)pandemic,England and Wales.* ONS. www.ons.gov.uk/peoplepopulationandcommunity/crimeand justice/articles/domesticabuseduringthecoronaviruscovid19pandemicengland andwales/november2020

Rosen, M.(2021). *Many different kinds of love.* Ebury Press.

For Liz's biographical details, see Chapter 1, p.39.

Resources

Mental and spiritual wellbeing

Books and articles

Bloom, A. (2022, April 2). After my husband died, my life felt broken – so I planted a new tree. *The Guardian.* www.theguardian.com/society/2022/apr/02/ amy-bloom-after-my-husband-died-my-life-felt-broken-so-i-planted-a-new-tree

Bloom, A. (2022). *In love: A memoir of love and loss*. Granta Books.

Cameron, J. (1992). *The artist's way: A spiritual path to higher creativity*. Profile Books.

Chatterjee, R. (2022). *Happy mind, happy life: 10 simple ways to feel great every day*. Penguin.

Chödrön, P. (2005). *When things fall apart: Heart advice for difficult times*. Harper.

Kabat-Zinn, J. (2014). *Mindfulness for beginners: Reclaiming the present moment and your life*. Sounds True.

Kimmerer, R.W. (2020). *Braiding sweetgrass*. Penguin.

Organisations and resources

Mental Health Foundation Covid Response Programme. Supporting lone parents, black and minority ethnic communities, refugees, and people with long term physical health conditions. *www.mentalhealth.org.uk/our-work/covid-response-programme*

National Council for Voluntary Organisations (NCVO). Finding the right volunteering role for you. *www.ncvo.org.uk/ncvo-volunteering/i-want-to-volunteer*

Arts and creativity

Big Brum Boogie Celebration. Flashmob dance created by students and care home residents with Autin Dance Theatre. (2021). *www.youtube.com/watch?v=tYfoG5H-7hI*

Grayson's Art Club. Grayson and Philippa Perry's Channel 4 series and online art club. *www.graysonsartclub.com*

Lockdown diaries. (2021). A part podcast and radio series from the Kashmiri Arts Heritage Foundation featuring short stories, poems and word-based anecdotes from Birmingham residents sharing their Covid experiences through creative writing. *www.lockdowndiariesbirmingham.com*

Notes from a Pandemic. Young Birmingham Poets (2022). For teachers – run your own reflective poetry project on the pandemic with your class. National Literacy Trust. *https://literacytrust.org.uk/communities/birmingham/schools/young-birmingham-poets-notes-from-a-pandemic*

Open Story Tellers. Supporting people with learning disabilities and autism to find their voice and use it. *www.openstorytellers.org.uk*

Stopgap Dance Company. Using dance as a movement for change and inclusivity. *https://www.stopgapdance.com*

Surviving through story: Living through the pandemic with learning disabilities. Open University project to collect and archive the stories of the lives of people with learning disabilities through the pandemic. *https://wels. open.ac.uk/news/surviving-through-story-living-through-pandemic-learning-disabilities*

The natural world, social change and climate justice

Reports and books

Climate Justice Alliance. (2020). *A people's orientation to a regenerative economy: Protect, repair, invest and transform.* Report. https://climatejusticealliance.org/regenerativeeconomy

Raworth, K .(2017). *Donut economics: Seven ways to think like a 21st century economist.* Random House.

Organisations and resources

Common Ground. Imaginative ways to connect people with their local environment. *www.commonground.org.uk*

Forest Schools. Fostering networks of educators working with children in outdoor classrooms. *www.forestschools.com*

Land Workers' Alliance. Union for people living on the land and growing food sustainably - farmers, growers, foresters and land-based workers, working for food sovereignty, sustainable forestry and the right to food. *https:// landworkersalliance.org.uk*

New Economics Foundation. Rethinking our economic goals and expectations. *https://neweconomics.org*

Ramblers. Opening the way for everyone to enjoy walking and protecting the places we love to wander. *www.ramblers.org.uk*

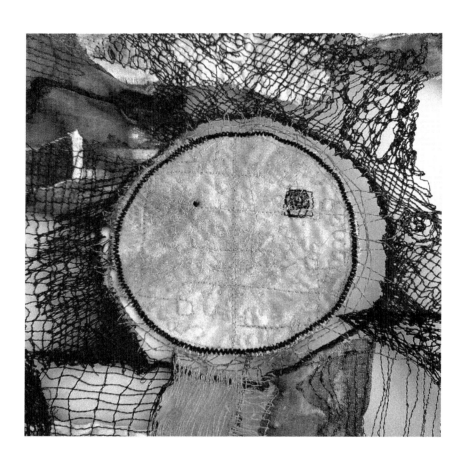

The Storytellers

With grateful thanks to all those who chose to withhold their names and so remain unmentioned but far from forgotten here.

Adam Hassan
Adele Moss
Ajeyar Madockhy
Alice Matthews
All is Mended Project
Amag Mardokhy
Amy Hodkin
Andrew Pennington
Andy
Andy Paine
Anita Luby
Anna
Avril Danczak
Barbara Welford
Basia Schofield
Bill Davis
Cally Ward
Carol Patton
Carole
Claire Bateman
Claire Hastie
Claire Stagg
Debbie Collins
Deborah Lewis
Diane Harris
Diane Pummell
Dionne Gbasai

Elaine Thorpe
Elizabeth Klyne
Ema
Emma
Emma Smith
Evie Moore
Fran Hall
Gordon Knott
Hannah Thomas
Hasina Zaman
Heidi Kennedy
Helen Chadwick
Iona Fabian
Irfan
Iulian Firea
Jackie Singer
Jacqui Alexander
Jacqui Kent
Jameisha Prescod
James Bailey
Jane
Jemima Meecham
Jeorgina Camelo
Jess Duckworth
Jo Goodman
John Pearce
Josie Webber

Joy Elliott
Jude Bishop
Julia
Julia Parker
Julia Samuel
Julie Kay
Katherine Brownlee
Katie Peacock
Kiera
Kiran Oram
Kristin Wallis
Laura Potts
Leshie Chandrapala
Libby Harris
Lily Howard
Limor
Linda
Lindsay Jackson
Liz
Liz Rothschild
Lucy Coulbert
Margaret Nairne
Marguerite Wallis
Maria
Marie Benham
Marie Francoise Rosat
Mary Maltby
Meredith Debonnaire
Michael and Esmay Rothschild
Nate Thompson
Nawaf
Nicky Hare
Pam Douglas
Paul Julian
Peter Burrows
Rahila Gupta
Rana Ibrahim
Rhys Wathen

Richard Benwell
Ruth Rosselson
Sally Hinchliff
Samir T
Sarah Anthony
Sarah Grylls
Sarah O'Connell
Sarah Pickthall
Sonia Oliver
Sophie Hunter
Sophie McManus
Sophy Thomas
Steph Muir
Steve Benham
Stuart Taylor
Susan
Thérèse Maitland
Tom Grant Edwards
Tomos Price
Tomos Williams
Tony
Trupti Magecha
Yansie Rolston
Yasotha Browne

The Artists

Tilly Cameron
Tilly is a multi-disciplinary artist currently based in Lincoln. Inspired by the life and work of Kurt Vonnegut, Margaret Atwood, Ruth Asawa, Diane Arbus, Austin Kleon, Chris McCandless, William Shakespeare and The Beatles to name but eight. www.popupartscollective.co.uk/tilly-cameron | tillycamerondevon2000@gmail.com

Clare Davis
Recapturing a dream of youth, Clare has become an exploratory artist in later life, working mainly in ink, wire and textile, and founder of the Pop Up Arts Collective. The collective is a diverse community of painters, sculptors, photographers, wordsmiths, makers and mixed media artists who have made a connection through family, friendship and creativity. They share a commitment to their artistic journeys, equality and access, and come together for workshops, creative conversations, residencies and exhibitions. Clare is a facilitator, mentor and tutor and works creatively with individuals and groups to encourage the creative flow, often working towards exhibition and communicating a story with a broad and dynamic approach to what art is and who artists are. www.popupartscollective.co.uk

Anna Dumitriu
Anna Dumitriu is an award-winning and internationally renowned British artist who works with BioArt, sculpture, installation and digital media to explore our relationship to infectious diseases, synthetic biology and robotics. Past exhibitions include ZKM, Ars Electronica, BOZAR, The Picasso Museum, HeK Basel, MOCA Taipei, Art Laboratory Berlin and Eden Project.

'Shielding' is impregnated with SARS-CoV-2 RNA (Coronavirus) from a plasmid construct. The piece is inspired by the hastily constructed temporary hospitals in Wuhan and Virginia Woolf's feminist text *A Room of One's Own* (1929). It explores the impact of lockdown on women facing domestic abuse and the paradoxical meaning of shelter. https://annadumitriu.co.uk

Ruby Frizell

I have always been around art and creativity. It has always surrounded me, so I couldn't say when I started creating, but I can say it has always been a constant. I've had mental health issues for four years, which partly stemmed from my struggles with school, where the environment was detrimental to me. So, honestly speaking, first going into lockdown was a relief for me, but that didn't take away the added confusion that Covid induced. My mum got me a sketch book and told me to use it to express what I couldn't with words. All the art I produced during that time, including my poetry and music, was also influenced by me being in love when the world was practically burning outside my window. Covid took so much from so many, but it allowed me to have time to do what I am truly passionate about.

Sarah Gillespie RWA

Born 1963, Sarah studied 15th- and 16th-century methods and materials at the Atelier Neo-Medici in Paris for one year before going on to Oxford University to read Fine Art at the Ruskin. She lives and works in Devon, specialising in drawing and mezzotint engraving, and is exhibited and collected by museums and individuals internationally. Most recently her entire Moth series has been acquired by the V&A Museum, London. She says of her work: 'My interest is in making an art that is emphatically not devoted to self-expression. In fact, I would like to dislodge the human-centered viewpoint from its pedestal and honour instead the fragile life of our fellow sentient beings – moths, trees, and birds. I believe the practice of paying attention to the more-than-human world to be the foundation of radical form of art. For me, to heed, to attend, to be "in conversation" with our fellow beings, to love and to allow ourselves to grieve for what is lost, is a practice that is at once devotional and subversive. We are not separate from our fellow beings; in fact, we are all quite literally made of the same stuff. We are relatives and share each other's fate.'

Wren Hughes is a sculptor and creative arts therapist whose work has been exhibited internationally over the last 40 years. The materials she uses varies from welded steel and stone to wax and bronze. Wren also draws, paints and uses mixed media. Her themes of death, transition and rebirth are an ongoing inquiry into the void and its significance in the creative process. Wren's retreats and contemplative art groups offer a combination of silence and creative exploration, a gentle invitation to live in the moment and trust what comes. www.wrenhughes.co.uk

Cath Jackson

Retired for many years from frontline cartooning, I was cajoled by Liz into picking up my pen again to contribute to this book. Now a wordsmith – editor and journalist, specialising in mental health and counselling.

Liz Rothschild

Not being able to find an image to fit this chapter in the way I imagined it, I turned to myself. I am not a trained visual artist, but I love playing with paper and pens and scissors when I get the chance, and hope to find more time in the future to do more of this.

Rowan Twine

Rowan is a behavioural insights researcher and part-time creator. Having explored cultures across two continents and three countries, she is currently based in Manchester, UK. People are at the centre of her work, and she is passionate about understanding them: both their relationships to each other and to their environments. She works across a range of mediums, returning most frequently to photography.

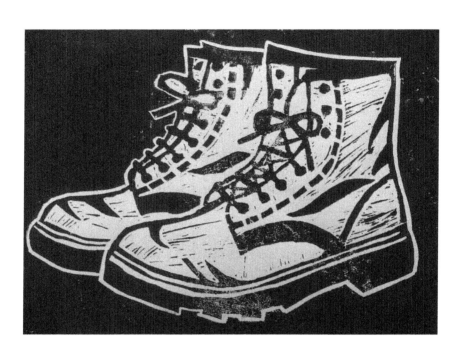